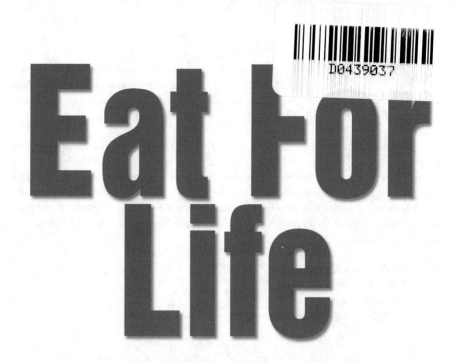

Eat For Life

THE ULTIMATE WEIGHT-LOSS BREAKTHROUGH

HARVEY DIAMOND

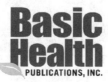

Basic Health
PUBLICATIONS, INC.

Basic Health Publications, Inc.
28812 Top of the World Drive
Laguna Beach, CA 92651
949-715-7327 • www.basichealthpub.com

Library of Congress Cataloging-in-Publication Data is available through the Library of Congress.

ISBN: 978-1-59120-305-6

Editor: Carol A. Rosenberg
Typesetting/Book design: Theresa Wiscovitch and Gary A. Rosenberg
Cover design: Mike Stromberg

Printed in the United States of America

10   9   8   7   6   5   4   3   2   1

CONTENTS

INTRODUCTION

HI, MY NAME IS HARVEY, AND OH BABY, do I love to eat. For as long as I can remember, sitting down to, or should I say diving into, some scrumptious meal of delectable food has always been right up there at the top of my "favorite things to do" list. Lots of people are ruled by their egos (or so I've heard). But me? I'm ruled by my taste buds. Being so enamored with food and its taste turns out to be a double-edged sword. On the one hand, food, in all of its glorious, lip-smacking diversity, has been an always-reliable source of pleasure and gratification. But then there's the flip side of all the gustatory indulgences: if one is not careful, that same source of so much pleasure can also be the source of pain, obesity, ill health, and even death.

I have wrestled with my weight for most of my adult life. Oddly, I was a *really* skinny kid. So much so, that other kids at school, and even my own brothers, made fun of me. Strangers tried to give me food! I'm serious. Until I was about eleven years old I grew up in a little coal-mining town called Harlan, Kentucky. Think of the fictional town of Mayberry as depicted on *The Andy Griffith Show* and you know what Harlan was like. In fact, that show could easily have been filmed in Harlan. Harlan was about as homey and laid back as any place you've ever seen. Everybody knew everybody else and friendliness was a way of life. You could knock on any door anywhere

1

in town and ask for some water because you were thirsty, some food because you were hungry, or even to use the bathroom, and you were invited in and treated like a long-lost cousin. I loved growing up there and have only the fondest memories of the place.

Harlanites would see me walking home from school and call me over and, after making some crack about my weight—like if I didn't put some rocks in my pocket a good wind was going to blow me away—they would ask, "Darlin', would you like a piece of cake?" Now what kid is going to turn down a piece a cake? But no matter how much I ate, I remained "skin and bones."

Even as a teenager, I never thought I would be fat. I had what I refer to as the "arrogance of the skinny." You know the types: eat as much of *anything* they like and never gain an ounce. Go to the beach and whip off their shirts with plenty of fanfare while looking around with pride to see if any of the ladies are watching. Not until I was in my late teens and early twenties did it start to become apparent to me that the party was over. It was a real shocker the first time I was forced to say to myself, "Hey, what's going on here? I'm getting chubby!" I actually went from someone who could completely throw caution to the wind and stuff myself with anything I pleased without gaining so much as a nanogram, to someone who put on weight by reading *Gourmet* magazine.

I spent four years in the military with my weight fluctuating up and down the entire time. My last year was in Vietnam where it could be 120 degrees for long stretches. Not only was the food not anything to write home about, but frequently the meals were "C" rations. If you like to eat, you don't want to know what "C" rations are. Here's a hint: they were left over from World War II! Between the stifling heat, the less than appetizing "regular" food, and the insufferable "C" rations, let's just say it was not a challenge to refrain from overeating. When I returned home in January 1967, I was 145 pounds. And that was the last time I was ever anywhere near that weight. My mom took one look at me, all emaciated and gaunt, and nearly fainted as she put her hands to her face and exclaimed, "Oh my God!" Her Jewish-mother thing kicked in and she started feeding me as if I were being fattened up for slaughter. I continued eating with wild abandon, and, well . . .

The next three and a half years were filled with anguishing over food, obsessing over my weight, and—one of my least favorite things to do in life—dieting. Lord, I hated to diet. But what else could I do if I didn't want to wind up blocking out the sun for my neighbors and having to grease my thighs to pass through a doorway? And I tried every whacked-out diet that appeared on the scene. Try eating celery and cottage cheese for thirty days straight and see how amiable you remain. Yes, I did do that one. Lost a lot of weight, too, but whoa, let's just say it was not fun. I always dieted for thirty days— don't know why exactly. It's just the number of days I convinced myself I had to do for it to be worthwhile. And I *would* lose weight.

For two days before I knew I would be going on a diet, I would stuff myself till food was oozing out of my ears, —making the first few days of the diet practically unbearable. Then I spent the remainder of the ordeal fantasizing over what foods I would ultimately gorge myself on when the agony of not being able to eat what I wanted was over.

Needless to say, I would always make all of these proclamations about how I was going to eat more healthfully and rationally after the diet was over, so I could maintain my weight loss and not have to diet anymore. Yeah, right. That lasted about a day and a half— maybe. After I fought mightily, and struggled and suffered to lose twenty-five or thirty pounds, which I always did, I wound up putting all the weight back on and then some. Back to square one, until I became so disgusted with myself that I went on the next diet that came along. No way to live.

DIETS DON'T WORK!

There are certain things in life that are self-evident. The sun is hot, and it's moist in the tropics—both self-evident; you don't need written proof. Politicians don't always tell the truth—again, self-evident. And there is something else that is patently self-evident: diets don't work! They are temporary measures that have failure built right into them. They are *designed* to fail. Because as soon as the diet is over and the old eating habits that brought on the need to diet in the first place return, all the weight comes back. Doing this over and over makes it harder and harder to lose the weight the next time. So in the long term, constant dieting will actually wind up making you heavier. How's that for irony?

I am closing in on my seventh decade on earth. I don't remember a time when diets were not in vogue. Have they worked? No! It's self-evident. About $60 billion is spent on weight loss a *year* in the United States alone. And what has that astounding expenditure of money reaped? After decades of dieting, we find ourselves today in the midst of the most dire obesity epidemic the world has ever known. It is now even affecting children in unprecedented numbers. That's some track record.

Do you think that over the *same* forty years during which wonder diets, weight-loss books, and other weight-loss schemes became popular that it is a mere coincidence that overweight and obesity have reached epidemic proportions? The reason why diets don't work long term is simple, really. Whether it's a diet from the past or one that is in vogue today, they *all* have the exact same shortcoming built into them that insures their long-term failure. All diets are designed, one way or another, with these four common goals: to help you lose *as much weight* as possible, *as fast* as possible, *by any means* possible, and *at any cost*!

Unfortunately, the single *most* important element required for *successful, long-term, permanent weight loss* is left out of this equation: how to so nourish and strengthen the body with proper diet that maintaining a healthy body weight becomes an *automatic* result of how and what you eat.

CHANGE YOUR "FOOD STYLE," CHANGE YOUR LIFE!

Did you know that today, while you are reading this book, 800 people will die of obesity-related causes? And 800 died yesterday, and another 800 will die tomorrow, and every day to follow if something isn't done to alter this sorrowful situation. Overweight and obesity contribute to such a wide range of ailments that I can't list them all here. Obesity is one of the officially designated five "diseases of afflu-ence" and is a major contributor to the *other* four: heart disease, can-cer, diabetes, and osteoporosis.

When it came to my own weight problem, I realized I couldn't continue going on and off diets. Not only is it depressing, but there is also evidence that doing so weakens the body overall. I had to make a change and figure out how to both enjoy eating *and* maintain my weight. In 1970 I was introduced to the 200-year-old field of "Natural Hygiene" (orthopathy), which relies on proper diet and nutrition in order to acquire *and* maintain an extremely high level of pain-free good health. I began to study the subject as though my life were at stake—as indeed it was! I learned that there was a way of eating that allowed for enjoying the eating experience while keeping my weight in check and supporting the body's natural effort to remain healthy. I never dieted again. Rather, I made some simple, yet enormously effective *permanent* dietary changes that became part of my lifestyle.

The result of my studies in the field of natural hygiene was the release of *Fit For Life* in 1985. The book became an instant sensa-tion, selling many millions of copies in thirty-four languages around the world. *Eat For Life* is my ninth book. Yes, it is a book about food and diet, but it is *not* a diet book.

Let me assure you that there is a humongous difference between "going on a diet" and "improving one's diet." Of course, you could say that unless you're not eating, *everyone* is on some kind of diet. Kind of a word play thing there, but I guess that's right. If you're eating, you're on a diet. But there are diets, and then there are *diets*. There are diets that suck the joy right out of eating (one of our most pleas-urable experiences), and there are diets that celebrate the *joys* of eat-ing. Guess which type I wish to present to you?

Perhaps a different mind-set is needed when it comes to "diets." Something like, "Yes, I'm on a diet, but not in the traditional sense.

Hey, I get to eat!" I want to rescue you from the type of dieting that breeds frustration and guilt. I want to rescue you from dieting as I have been rescued, by introducing you to two means by which you can stop those restricted, regimented diets that ultimately end with disappointment. Instead, you can be on a diet that will help you lose weight *and* enjoy eating, with no deprivation, no calorie counting, no portion measuring, no chalky-tasting meal-replacement drinks—and none of the other annoying aspects of dieting that turn the eating experience into a clinical exercise. Sound good?

YOUR FIRST TOOL FOR ULTIMATE WEIGHT LOSS: ENZYMES!

The first means by which you can lose weight without dieting involves using a specially formulated enzyme product. It is not often that I am so bowled over by a genuinely top-notch product that can do so much good for so many people that I want to shout its praises from the mountaintop. The last time I was this excited was in 1995 when I was introduced to *supplemental* digestive enzymes, an entirely natural product that streamlines and enhances the activities of the digestive tract to increase energy and reduce stomach and digestive ailments. From that day until now I have been taking digestive enzymes, without fail, whenever I eat anything that's been cooked, and they have been a real blessing in my life.

Well, here I am inspired to start shouting again, and wouldn't you know it, it's another enzyme product. Yes, it is a completely natural, highly effective enzyme blend that assists the body in losing weight: Slender GR™.

Now, before going one word further, I must address something. I know there is bound to be someone at least a little familiar with *Fit For Life* who is going to ask, "Hey, aren't you the guy who admonished me not to seek remedies in a bottle?" Yup, that's me. So why am I now endorsing that very thing?

In every area of life, great leaps and bounds have been made over the years since the release of *Fit For Life*. As one obvious example, consider the World Wide Web; it didn't even exist when that book was written. Or think of cell phones, which are ubiquitous and something we take for granted; back then if your car broke down on the highway, you had to hike to a phone booth to call for help. Similarly, in the arena of diet and health, great strides have been made in the growing, harvesting, extraction, formulation, and delivery of vital nutrients. And nothing more profoundly illustrates that fact than the revolutionary process that brings to consumers an array of highly effective enzyme products that work in harmony with the body.

What is exciting about Slender GR™ is that it succeeds in helping you lose weight *without* the dangerous, sometimes deadly, side effects routinely associated with pharmaceuticals. Periodically we see much hoopla and fanfare related to the latest attempt to market a weight-loss drug like Fen-Phen, Meridia, Metabolife, Xenical, and Qnexa. But invariably, the side effects keep them from being approved for sale. I'm not only talking about the standard side effects of headache, stomachache, dizziness, nausea, and the like, I'm referring to the real drawback with these drugs: increased blood pressure, heart disease, stroke, kidney and pancreas problems, and even death! No matter how badly people wish to lose weight I don't think they're willing to put their lives at stake to do so.

In addition, there are other "fat-burning" supplements on the market (called "thermogenics"), which are designed to increase metabolism and suppress appetite by using stimulants such as caffeine and ephedrine—both associated with irregular heartbeat, insomnia, and elevated blood pressure.

What sets Slender GR™ apart from all such products associated with weight loss is the fact that it is a completely harmless, totally natural substance derived entirely from living plant sources, with no unsafe or hurtful ingredients, no synthetics, and no foreign, chemical additives of any kind. Rather than trying to force or trick the body into losing weight with artificial stimulants or chemicals, Slender

GR™ works in harmony *with* the body to bring about weight loss. If this were not so, I would not be as excited about it nor would I be attaching my name to its unveiling.

It is important for you to know that some exceptionally knowledgeable people in the world of enzymes—who have an abiding commitment to giving you something pure and effective that will help you, not hurt you—have worked diligently to bring this innovative and groundbreaking product to you.

Chapter 2 reveals some basic information about what enzymes are and the monumental, incomparable role they play in everyone's life. Later in the book, Dr. Steven Lamm will give details on what Slender GR™ is, how it works in the body, and what you can expect from its use.

For now, just to end a little of the suspense, allow me to give you a short and simple description of how Slender GR™ succeeds in helping you lose weight. First, as you may or may not already know (my guess is you do), the human body is an amazingly efficient fat-storing machine. It's all tied into survival—the body wants to keep fat reserves on hand that might be needed at a later date should the body be deprived of food. This explains those survival stories we've all heard about people being stranded in the wilderness for ten, twenty, even thirty days or more with some water, but no food whatsoever. When they're rescued, aside from having lost weight and being somewhat dehydrated and exhausted, they are in surprisingly good shape. They survived on their fat reserves. (And no, I'm not going to introduce you to the "Wilderness Diet.")

Every activity of the body, large or small, requires energy, and in the absence of sufficient carbohydrates, fat will be burned for energy. So think of body fat as a sort of emergency storage reservoir for energy, should it be needed. Now, of course, some fat reserves are important—in fact, very important. The idea that fat is evil and we must rid ourselves of every last trace of it is patently absurd. We need a certain amount of fat to survive. But let's face it, because of an inferior diet resulting in poor nutrition, coupled with a sedentary lifestyle consisting of too little physical exercise, these reserves have gotten way out of hand and are far in excess of what the body needs to take care of itself. What the body needs to normalize fat reserves *and* to take care of *all* bodily needs is energy, and energy is tied into the body's metabolism.

You likely know what the word *metabolism* means. However, just to be sure we're on the same wavelength, here is a simple, straightforward description: Metabolism is the entire range of biochemical activities that take place within the living body to convert food into energy and the other substances necessary for life. Metabolism utilizes enzymes that transform one substance into another substance. That's it.

Slender GR™ contains two primary enzymes that assist the body in ridding itself of excess fat. The first is lipase (words that end with "ase" are types of enzymes), which is the enzyme that breaks down fat. It turns out that there are those who have a genetic lipase deficiency and therefore struggle with weight loss since the body, as we know, has a tendency to store fat. One study showed that 100 percent of clinically obese people (over 30 percent above their ideal body weight) were lipase deficient. The additional lipase provided by Slender GR™ helps balance any deficiency, which results in both more efficient letting go of excess stored fat *and* increased fat metabolism—a good combination if weight loss is one of your goals.

I'm not one for bogging down my readers with a bunch of incomprehensible jargon and technical, scientific descriptions, so the name of the second ingredient in—Slender GR™ Glucoreductase™ (GR) —might at first blush look like one of those baffling, multisyllabled words you can throw a saddle on and ride around the backyard. But it's really not. The first part of the word is derived from the word *glucose* (gluco), the second part from the word *reduce* (reduct), and the third part means enzyme (ase).

Slender GR's™ second ingredient, Glucoreductase™ is actually a blend of several enzymes that convert simple sugars into fiber. This action lowers what is referred to as the caloric value of carbohydrates and provides a food source for naturally occurring microflora in the body. This, in turn, results in a reduction of insulin demand. Insulin is a hormone secreted by your pancreas. It assists in transporting glucose in your blood (or blood sugar) into your cells where it is converted into fuel. Why is reduced insulin demand so important in terms of losing weight? Because high insulin demand, and output, signals the body to store fat. So the enzyme Glucoreductase™ actually reduces the amount of sugar that enters the bloodstream, thereby lowering demand for insulin production and reducing stored fat.

YOUR SECOND TOOL FOR ULTIMATE WEIGHT LOSS: ALTERING WHAT, WHEN, AND HOW YOU EAT

The second tool I'll share with you to help you lose weight consists of some extremely simple dietary tips from my Fit For Life program that you can use, according to your own comfort level, in order to increase the effectiveness of Slender GR™ as well as your overall health and well-being. I want you to know that these dietary guidelines are time-tested, tried, and proven—they work! Millions of people will attest to that statement. The principles of eating delineated in the *Fit For Life* books have been remarkably successful for people over the years, and it is from these books that I have extracted a few of the basics to help you in your quest.

Let me be crystal clear about something here. When I say I'm going to share some dietary tips to help you, some may immediately think, *Oh, here it comes. Tips my foot—probably more like rules that will have me eating nothing but alfalfa sprouts and shredded carrots three days a week.* I want to allay any such concerns and tell you that the dietary tips I will share are *not* required for you to have results while taking Slender GR™. In fact, data collected from the study group involved in testing the effectiveness of Slender GR™ showed that even those who made no dietary changes whatsoever still lost weight. However, the weight loss experienced with Slender GR™ can be maximized with these dietary tips, which have been designed to help you increase the effectiveness of the enzyme while allowing you to enjoy the eating experience. And I am confident that once you see how truly simple *and* effective my dietary tips are, you will *want* to make use of them.

It's such an interesting phenomenon to me that I have seen time and again over the years; as soon as the subject of diet is raised people start to place far too many restrictions and demands on themselves and confine themselves to this "either-or" scenario. And with the *slightest* digression, they are in turmoil; berating themselves: "I'm worthless, I can't stick to anything!" Then it's off to some bingeing to make the point, which only serves to make themselves feel even worse about their situation. This is especially true if they are following a prescribed diet. It's as though their mindset is locked into the whole reward/punishment model and they have no "wiggle room". "Ooh if I'm good I'll lose that weight; if I'm not I'm going to suffer."

I want to tell you something—fanaticism does not work. Not in politics, not in religion, and not with diet. Fanaticism just makes things worse in the long run. That's why it is extremely important you understand that the simple dietary tips I will be sharing with you are *not* inflexible rules. They are designed to help you increase the effectiveness of Slender GR™ while allowing you to enjoy the eating experience.

It's like this; right now the price of gas is ridiculously high. For some people it is the biggest expenditure right behind rent and food. Consequently, people are taking measures to use less gas by driving less, carpooling, and driving in a manner that conserves rather than squanders gas. Gone are the days when ten bucks would fill your gas tank—twice! Now you know how old I am for sure. One can conserve gas by not taking off from the standing position by lurching forward quickly but rather gradually, driving at a steady speed, and not "flooring it" to change lanes up and back. That's a reasonable, gas-saving way to drive. But you know what? Sometimes you are going to drive like that, high gas prices or not; either because you're late for something important, like a business appointment, or picking up your kid from school, or trying to get to the airport on time for a flight. If it's convenient to drive leisurely, well, it just makes good sense to do so and save gas, right? If it's not convenient, then it's not, that's all there is to it—you do what you have to do and move on.

I don't know if that's the best analogy but that's how it is with the dietary tools I will be sharing with you. If my dietary tips and tools are convenient for you, fine; if not, also fine. So there doesn't ever have to be anything like, "Uh oh, I had a bite of cinnamon toast—I'm doomed." You'll see—it's very relaxed and freeing. And why should the atmosphere around food and eating be otherwise? It's a part of life we love!

There's an old saying most people are familiar with: "If it ain't broke, don't fix it." That's how I feel about the dietary principles in *Fit For Life* that have helped so many people around the world. That does not mean that they cannot be adapted to accommodate those people who, for whatever reason, can or will not use them the way they are presented or, despite doing so, are not satisfied with the results. No matter what anyone tells you, no one approach to diet is right for everyone. People have genetic differences, and that's just a fact of life.

There are those whose metabolism is highly efficient while there are others whose metabolism is "sluggish." Some people have digestive shortcomings or naturally occurring food sensitivities or blood sugar issues or any number of other variables at work that make the "one-size-fits-all" idea to diet unrealistic. And yes, that includes *Fit For Life*. True, most people who eat according to the principles laid out in my books are successful in losing weight if that is their desire, but I can also tell you of those who didn't. In one instance, a woman told me that even though she and her husband followed *Fit For Life* to the letter and supported one another in doing so, he lost 35 pounds and she did not lose an ounce. And I can tell you of another instance where it was the opposite; the wife lost weight and the husband didn't.

One thing that comes with circling the sun as many times as I have is the understanding that comes with experience. I have no problem acknowledging the fact that notwithstanding what I have learned over the years, it is but a fraction of what is yet to be learned that resides in what I like to call the "Great Unknown." After more than forty years of study, I am *still* studying and learning, and I pray to the powers that be that I never stop learning new and innovative ideas and truths that, in some cases, may render obsolete the past beliefs I strongly held.

I know of contemporaries of mine—two that I am thinking of in particular-whose names will remain unspoken, who are brilliant researchers and teachers who have helped millions of people, including me. But they have become so set in their thinking and beliefs, convinced that they know what there is to know in their area of expertise, that any disagreement or challenge to their think-ing, no matter how minute, valid or not, is met with anger and vit-riol. It is as though any difference of opinion is viewed as an attack on their person. I would never want to be so intractable that such a thing would be said about me. Anyone can proudly declare that they are right; it takes a much bigger, stronger person to declare that they are wrong.

My point here is that there are people who want to use the prin-ciples of *Fit For Life* but for whatever reason, can't fit them into their lifestyle. So if I have to alter the material somewhat, or make an allowance for these people, or make an exception for them, I will. Some who read this book who are familiar with *Fit For Life* will find information that will be like a refresher course for them; some will see what appears to be an inconsistency with what they have read in the past, which is actually my effort to modify the information somewhat in order to make it useful to everyone. Why should anyone be left out of using information that can help them look and feel better? Those of you for whom this information is brand new, may it be a revelation in your life as it has been for so many others.

THE TWO-PRONGED APPROACH FOR ULTIMATE WEIGHT LOSS

I feel enormously confident that if you try Slender GR™ and utilize the dietary principles that support its effectiveness, you will be supremely gratified. Now, as someone familiar with the mentality of those who want to lose weight, I know that perhaps the first question on your lips is, "How much weight will I lose and how long will it take?" See? I told you I knew what you were thinking.

Aside from the fact that there are regulatory agencies that prohibit making claims about how much weight you will lose by taking a certain product, it's not very realistic to categorically state how much will be lost. I've seen ads, as I'm sure you have, that make all sorts of unrealistic, outlandish claims in order to sell a product. They like to leave you with the idea that all you have to do is take a certain pill before you go to sleep at night and you will wake up in the morning needing to buy a new wardrobe because your weight magically melted away. You know deep down that's a load of pony loaf.

Most claims about immediate, significant loss of weight are made by people who lost water. Hey, lots of people can show you how to lose a bunch of weight in a few days by dehydrating yourself. There are athletes—boxers, wrestlers, MMA fighters, and bodybuilders— who will, in order to make a certain weight class, lose 15 pounds in a couple of days. So what? At what cost? And it certainly isn't permanent. What I can assure you is that what I want, and what the developer of Slender GR™ wants—first and foremost—is to provide you with something that does not put your health at risk. Any diet designed to lose weight that is not nutritionally sound is going to fail you in the long term.

I'm sure it's a pretty good bet that if you are trying to lose weight it's not something you have been dealing with for weeks or months, but rather years. Am I right? Let me give you something realistic to consider. First, know that removing excess fat from your body is not like losing water. Water can be dropped in significant amounts relatively quickly. But as it happens, actual fat is removed from the body rather slowly; it's the nature of how the body works.

What if you could *safely* lose 1½ to 2 pounds a week? Would that interest you? Now, if you have 30 or 40 or more extra pounds you're toting around you might be thinking, *Hey, that's bupkis.* But 1½ to 2 pounds a week translates to 6 to 8 pounds a month. That means in only four months time you could lose 24 to 32 pounds. Now that's the kind of real expectation I want you to have.

YOUR AMAZING BODY

Before bringing this introduction to a close, I would like to leave you with one more enormously encouraging bit of information. You have the most dependable and capable ally in existence to assist you in realizing your most cherished health goals: your own body. That's right. Don't chuckle or make light of that statement. I know that when you're frustrated because you can't lose weight or you can't get into that swimsuit you want to wear, or you're not feeling well because of some pain or discomfort, or any number of other challenges associated with your body, it's easy to view your body as your enemy. Nothing could be further from the truth.

Make no mistake about it; the greatest, most brilliant minds the world has ever known are to this day bewildered and perplexed by what the living human body is capable of doing with seeming ease. There are those in the scientific community the world over who are convinced that the full measure of the intelligence governing the living body will never, ever be fully understood. The body is capable of performing tasks in such prodigious numbers, and with such perfection, that even to try to comprehend it all is an exercise in futility.

Just as an example, the body continuously, without letup or rest, pumps six quarts of blood through over 60,000 miles of blood vessels, bringing oxygen that it picked up from the lungs to every one of the *trillions* of cells in the body. It does this while maintaining a steady temperature, while maintaining balance, while coordinating more than 200 bones and more than 600 muscles in order to enable you to move in any direction you wish at anytime you wish. And this is but a mere *fraction* of what the body is doing every moment of every day and night.

I could easily go on and on describing with superlatives the incomprehensible intelligence that governs *your* living body, but let me just mention two more that pretty much stuns the intellect of anyone who contemplates these matters.

Imagine, if you will, gathering in one room the most exceptionally gifted and highly accomplished scientists in the world—the smartest, the brightest, the best of the best. If they were handed an apple and asked to turn it into human blood they would look at you like you had taken leave of your senses. Even given access to the most sophisticated, cutting-edge laboratory equipment in existence they could no more turn an apple, or any other food for that matter, into blood than they could sprout wings, fly to the moon, pick up a few handfuls of dust, and then fly back to earth and sprinkle it on your houseplants. And yet, with apparent ease, the living body not only turns apples and other foodstuffs into blood, it also turns it into bone, skin, teeth, hair, organs—anything it needs anytime it is needed. And no one knows how the body does this. Stunning!

Let us consider the human brain. Many scientists who have dedicated their lives to studying the human brain are firmly convinced that the true magnificence of this astonishing marvel of creation will never be fully understood. The study of the brain has been likened to the study of the cosmos. As much as is known of this remarkable organ—and it is considerable—it is still considered to be in the embryonic stages of understanding.

To give you a mere glimmer of the mind-boggling ability of the brain, consider this: There are approximately 7 billion inhabitants on earth. In today's climate of strife and turmoil, imagine all 7 billion acting and thinking harmoniously in complete unison. As absurd as such a suggestion is, compared to what the brain is doing *every moment* that's nothing!

There are 100 trillion cells in the human body. That's a one with fourteen zeros! Every one of these hundred trillion cells is constantly sending messages to the brain asking for instructions, and remarkably, the brain receives and answers each one—*simultaneously*! We're not talking about *seven* billion; we're talking about *one hundred thousand* billion, all working in complete harmony with one another with the brain at the helm! These trillions of messages are sent up and back twenty-four hours a day—ceaselessly coordinating and directing the countless functions of the body with absolute precision, and if need be, will continue doing so for a hundred years or more!

Only with such staggering images as these is it possible to have some sense of what the human brain is capable of achieving. It's been said that to even begin to comprehend the magnitude of the brain's splendor we would have to possess an intellect infinitely more developed than it is at present. We should be in a constant state of astonishment over our bodies, yet we take them largely for granted.

And you, my fortunate friend, have one of these astounding machines working on your behalf *every* moment! And guess what your body's number-one priority is? Your health and well-being! You should be jumping up and down with excitement and high-fiving the person nearest to you. Your remarkably intelligent body, with capabilities that baffle all of science, is *always* striving, tirelessly, to correct *anything* in need of repair; it's hardwired into the very core of the living body's survival mechanism.

Be very clear about something; the living body is self-repairing, self-healing, and self-maintaining. As an obvious example, just think of a cut finger—what do you think heals up a wound should you cut yourself? The Band-Aid? Hardly. The intelligent body immediately snaps into action and does what is necessary to heal the wound. And that is exactly what it does if there is something compromising your health and well-being *anywhere* in your body; it snaps into action and goes about fixing it as quickly and efficiently as possible and there's nothing in all of existence that can rival its ability to do so.

Whether it's an obstruction that needs to be cleared, an organ that needs to be repaired, toxins that need to be cleansed, or excess fat that needs to be removed, the intelligent body knows exactly what is going on and will go about the business of doing whatever needs to be done to remedy the situation. And all it needs from you is a little support and cooperation; it needs you to get out of its way and allow it to unleash its awesome, incomparable healing powers. Regarding your effort to lose weight, between taking Slender GR™ and following the simple dietary guidelines you will learn throughout this book, you will have the tools you need to provide your body with that support and cooperation.

I wish you success in this, and in all the endeavors of your life.

1

DOES HEAT MAKE YOU FAT?

CLEARING UP CALORIE
CONFUSION

You might be asking yourself right now, What does Harvey mean by "Does heat make you fat?" How in the world can heat make you fat? If heat makes you fat, I think that people living in close proximity to the equator would be a pretty hefty bunch. But as it happens, people living on or near the equator are the opposite: they're more on the lean side. So what am I even getting at here?

Do you happen to be a member of the group that thinks calories make you fat? And that the more calories you consume the fatter you become? (Unless, of course, you manage to burn them off.) Let me ask you this: do you know precisely what a calorie is? If someone asked you to define the word "calorie," could you easily and clearly give an accurate definition? Try it. Randomly ask people to tell you what a calorie is. Most will say something like, "Those things that make you fat, right?" The more clever might say, "Yeah, they're those sneaky little characters that slip into your closet at night and restitch your clothing to make it too small."

Allow me to give you the simplest and most succinct definition of a calorie: A calorie is a measure of heat. In point of fact, a calorie measures how much heat is required to raise the temperature of one gram of water by one degree centigrade. That's it. That's not conjecture, nor is it open for discussion or interpretation.

So . . . how has heat (calories) become the villain in the whole weight-loss thing? I don't know. I really don't. People have been counting calories for as long as I can remember. Has it done any good? It sure doesn't seem like it has, considering that people count calories like mad and the population is as overweight as ever—in fact, more so. This is an enormously controversial subject. There are people—weight-loss experts—who are convinced beyond any possible doubt that the only way to successfully lose weight is to count calories unfailingly: measure how many go in and how many go out and, depending upon which amount exceeds the other, you gain or lose weight. Eat more than you burn off and you will gain weight; burn off more than you eat and you will lose weight. Actually, it all seems reasonable enough to me.

But then there are other people—*also* weight-loss experts—who are just as convinced that the entire calorie-counting thing is a complete waste of time. They point out that merely keeping count of how many calories you consume in a day oversimplifies the complex nature of the body and how food is broken down and ultimately used as energy. Also, the composition of calorie sources varies dramatically. These experts point out that most people haven't the vaguest idea how many calories they should consume a day. That's because there are variables that come into play for different individuals. People's weight and size, their age, their sex, their level of physical activity, and more, can cause calorie requirements to vary dramatically.

Other experts point out that calories are *not* our enemy but, in fact, are our friends. After all, they provide the energy we need to fuel the numerous activities of the body. You certainly wouldn't say that gasoline is the enemy of cars, would you? Gasoline fuels cars and they couldn't run without some in the tank. Well, calories are to humans what gasoline is to cars. Calories are our fuel. If you put the wrong fuel in your car it won't run properly. In fact, the wrong fuel may very well destroy the engine. The same holds true with our bodies. Yes, we must take in fuel (calories), but it has to be the *right* fuel. And when one considers how long the issue of calories has been a central talking point in the discussion of fat and weight loss, and the obvious fact that overweight and obesity remains a significant problem, I'd say that it's not just merely the number of calories going into the body but also the *source* of the food delivering the calories. This all seems reasonable to me because a hundred years or so of counting calories sure hasn't resulted in all the desired weight loss. All indications are that the opposite is true.

And please don't think for a moment that the controversy over whether or not calories help or hinder the effort to shed weight is a new one. Consider the words of Phillip N. Norman, M.D., in 1924: "The conception of the calorie has retarded logical and rational reasoning in regard to diet, more than any other single factor." Wow! In 1924 they were arguing over the issue of calories, and the debate continues to be waged today, so many decades later. Both schools of thought seem to make valid points, quite frankly, which is why I find it somewhat disconcerting when one side or the other make these uncompromising, absolute statements supporting their positions while declaring that anyone who thinks otherwise is a moron. It's not as though anyone could actually have *all* the answers on a subject that is so obviously fraught with different, reasonably sounding positions.

CALORIES IN, CALORIES OUT? REALLY?

There are medically credentialed, conventional scientist types who persist in clinging to the "a calorie is a calorie is a calorie" mind-set. Their contention, backed up by their scientific background, is that when it comes to calories, it's "calories in versus calories out," so the *only* criteria for removing excess fat from the body is that as long as more calories leave the body than enter the body, fat will be lost *irrespective* of the source of the calories. In other words, take in 2,500 calories, from *any* source, and burn off 3,000 calories, and fat will be lost. Positions like that make me leery of people who smugly wave their credentials in your face as a means of certifying their argument. As though a piece of paper on the wall automatically confers upon the holder some proof of their intelligence and validates their position.

I'll tell you what I like to do when confronted with people who dictatorially insist that a "calorie is a calorie is a calorie" and to think otherwise is "unscientific." I challenge them to a little real-life experiment. We will both eat exactly 2,500 calories a day for one month. S/he will eat *only* potato chips and candy bars, and I will eat *only* fresh fruit and salad. So far, no one has taken me up on the challenge. In fact, the challenge is customarily met with derision and the entire idea waved off as ludicrous. They tell me I'm merely grandstanding. But when I push it and make it clear I'm dead serious, some statement is made about such a ridiculous test not proving anything, and besides, "You're not even a doctor!"

My point is that the subject of calories, like so many other areas in the vast arena of diet and health, is not always so cut and dry that there is no room for different points of view. Other factors come into play that must be considered. I will share one more revealing incident with you on this subject that I think makes the point well about the nature of calories and taking a position thereafter that is unassailable.

Five years before the release of *Fit For Life,* a most popular diet book of the day was *The Rotation Diet* by Dr. Martin Katahn, who was director of the Weight Management Program at Vanderbilt University. He was very well respected and his diet was based on calorie counting: calories in, calories out. Well, ten years later he came out with another diet book called *The T-Factor Diet,* the "T" representing the "thermogenic" effect of burning up calories for energy. His contention, which quickly caught on and was roundly praised, was that carbohydrate calories are burned faster and more efficiently than fat calories. What he was able to show was that calories derived from fat hung around on the body longer than calories derived from carbohydrates. In other words, in his newer book, he proved that the assertion he made in his previous book of "a calorie is a calorie is a calorie" was false. Oops.

But you have to give credit where credit is due—Dr. Katahn did the honorable thing and opened his new book with a message to the reader declaring that based on further research and knowledge, he realized that many of the old ideas about the caloric value of foods to the human body were wrong. In part, he stated, "All calories are not the same to the human body. When it comes to being overly fat or overweight, it's primarily the fat calories that count, not the carbohydrate and protein calories."

SCIENCE VERSUS SCIENCE FICTION

Part of what creates confusion in the public's mind when it comes to diet, health, and losing weight is the overabundance of divergent, opposing views on what's best. And contributing mightily to that confusion are all the experts who are quick to point out scientifically sound studies that reinforce and validate their particular premise. The only problem with that, and I hope this doesn't come off as *too* cynical, is the fact that unfortunately we live in an era when, depending upon who is conducting the study—and more important, who is *funding* the study—just about any premise can be proven.

I could easily write a big, fat chapter delineating the abundance of some of the more outrageous claims "proven" by scientific authorities that were later revealed to be, let us say, hogwash. In fact, one need look no further than the head of cancer research at the American Medical Association (AMA) testifying before Congress in 1957, using all of the latest scientific data, to reveal that "cigarette smoking is a harmless habit up to twenty-four cigarettes a day," and that "a pack a day keeps lung cancer away." No, I'm not kidding—Google it! Just as an interesting aside, the two men, both avid smokers, responsible for this remarkably off-the-mark bit of "science" were Dr. Ian McDonald and Dr. Henry Garland, two well-respected, upstanding medical doctors. Dr. McDonald incinerated himself in a fire started by the cigarette he was holding when he fell asleep, and Dr. Garland died of—you guessed it—lung cancer. Hey, you can't make this stuff up.

I will share with you my all-time favorite example of two scientifically sound studies proving opposite premises to be true. The reason it is the one I like to refer to the most is because the studies weren't in some obscure, second- or third-tier journal no one has even heard of. They were published in what many consider to be one of the premier, most highly respected medical journals in the world: *The New England Journal of Medicine.* Not only did the two studies appear in this prestigious journal, they were published in *the same issue!* One study "proved" that hormone replacement therapy (HRT) dramatically *increased* heart attacks in postmenopausal women; the other "proved" that HRT dramatically *decreased* heart attacks. This was so blatantly incongruous that the editor of the journal was compelled to write a letter to the reader explaining that both studies were impeccably conducted so both merited being published.

By no means am I trying to imply that there are no honestly conducted, worthwhile studies whose results can be depended upon. There are. By the same token, there are some that are not dependable, and they can definitely cloud the waters. I think the point I am trying to make here is clear. The next time someone declares to you, "This is how it is and here are the studies to prove it," perhaps you will recall what you have read here and at least consider the fact that "It ain't necessarily so." The subject of diet and health is rarely either black or white with no shades of gray.

Look, obviously something is up with the issue of calories being involved with eating, energy, and weight gain and loss. And maybe I'm just getting hung up on semantics because the actual meaning of the word "calorie" is *heat.* Perhaps if calories were called "units of energy" I would be having an easier time with the issue. It's not as though calories are little balls of fat that enter the body and make a beeline for the belly and thighs. And I'm not trying to claim or convince you that I have all the answers regarding calories and our weight, because I don't. I'm trying to understand it same as you. What I'm trying to say is that if someone did have all the answers and had it all figured out, we wouldn't still be shelling out $60 billion a year trying to get our weight under control, would we?

What has helped me most over the years in figuring out the best course of action healthwise is relying on common sense and experience. After all, you don't really have to be a highly credentialed scientist to know that you're going to fare a lot better and have an easier time maintaining your weight and your overall well-being on a healthy diet of fruit and vegetables than on an unhealthy diet of potato chips and candy bars. Clearly, I know that neither of these two extremes is realistic, but I'll bet there aren't too many people who would have any doubts whatsoever as to which of these two extremes would be better if they were forced to make a choice.

That being the case, common sense tells me two things. First, the diet that *would* be realistic is going to fall somewhere between the two extremes. Second, if whole, natural, unprocessed fruits and salads would be the unanimous choice over highly processed, devitalized, chemical-laden potato chips and candy bars, then it stands to reason that the closer your diet is to the healthier of the two options the better. *How* close is open for discussion, but no one who is serious about his or her health is going to opt for a diet that offers no nutrition and contributes to overweight and ill health.

What would be prudent to do is find those areas in which there is the greatest degree of agreement among people and allow those areas to be the guiding principles. There are certain aspects of this entire discussion that enjoy general unanimity among people. It is when determining the specifics within those generalities that differences of opinion tend to arise.

THE REAL "SCIENCE" AROUND FOOD: PROTEINS, FATS, AND CARBOHYDRATES

No one disputes the fact that we must eat food to live and that the three primary classifications of food are proteins, fats, and carbohydrates. No one disputes the fact that it is from those three food classes that the body must extract the two things it requires in order to stay alive—nutrients and an energy source.

As stated earlier, the living human body is an awesome machine, and its absolute, number-one priority is to stay alive. In order to do so it *must* extract from food the nutrients it needs to carry out the countless activities necessary to prolong life *and* an energy source to fuel those activities. Somewhere within that dynamic of taking in food, extracting and assimilating what the body needs from that food, and removing the waste that is generated in the process is where problems arise, be it excess weight or illness—along with differences of opinion on why and how to remedy those situations.

The entirety of nature in all its glorious magnificence is unfolding with a flawless precision and elegance that we cannot even comprehend. There is nothing in all of nature that is arbitrary or haphazard. From the farthest reaches of the cosmos in which we live, down to the structure of the atom, and everything in between, the exactness and intricacy of the natural world staggers the intellect and leaves all who study the sciences in humbled awe.

There is an infinite, incomprehensible intelligence at work in the universe that has created and governs all that exists, *and it knows what it is doing.* We can only stand as witnesses and marvel at its indescribable precision. The Moon circles the Earth, which in turn circles the Sun, with a mathematical exactness that is unwavering. A seed put into the ground will interact with the soil, water, and air and grow into a majestic 200-foot sequoia tree or a delicate orchid that dazzles the eye. This and more than can be described are all orchestrated by the limitless intelligence of which I speak.

This intelligence has also worked out what it is that we humans need to eat on a regular basis in order to remain alive and well. Could anyone possibly think it is an accident or some random occurrence that there are three categories of food that make up the human diet? Not four, not two, but *three:* proteins, fats, and carbohydrates. There's nothing haphazard about this; it is by design! One category is no more or less important than any other one. It is when *all three* are consumed, in the proper balance, and in the purest form, of course, that the body can excel at its highest level of health possible.

Let's briefly look at the three categories and see what purpose each fulfills.

❏ **Proteins.** Proteins are used for the building, repairing, and maintenance of all living tissue.

❏ **Fats.** Fats are used for insulation against heat loss; padding and protection for the organs; and as regulators of the fat-soluble vitamins A, D, E, and K.

❏ **Carbohydrates.** The purpose of carbohydrates in the human diet is for fuel energy. That's it. They have no other purpose. Carbohydrates equal energy—you know, that stuff we need every day in order to stay alive and carry out the uncountable activities performed by the human body day in and day out. Interestingly, there is not a single living thing on Earth that does not contain carbohydrates. Life would cease to exist without them.

To arbitrarily defy the grand scheme of life—to in effect try to thwart the infinite intelligence of the universe that carefully worked out this majestic plan—and either remove entirely one of these categories for *any* reason, or suggest that one is somehow inferior to the others, displays an arrogance and disdain for the natural order of things that defies all reason and is, quite frankly, counterproductive.

Why Diets Fail: Flying in the Face of Nature

A primary reason why so many classic diets fail in the long term is because of this ill-advised defiance of the natural, interconnected nature of food and its role in our well-being. There are high-protein diets that severely restrict or remove almost all carbohydrates. There are high-carbohydrate diets that severely restrict or remove almost all protein. Such diets fly in the face of natural law and doom themselves to failure.

Do you know what the living body is always striving for in all things? Homeostasis—balance! From an individual cell, to the entire natural world, to the health of the planet itself, balance is central to survival. The idea of trying to circumvent this fundamental tenet of life by restricting or removing one of the three vital elements of food and then counting calories to make up for it is laughable.

One extremely popular diet advises unlimited amounts of protein and the nearly total exclusion of carbohydrates. According to this diet you could sit down to a meal of a pound of butter deep-fried in bacon grease and top it off with a big slice of lard pie. But eat so much as a single grape and you're done for. The author of this insane approach to diet has managed to convince people that carbohydrates are evil. I will discuss the entire sugar/carbohydrate issue in a later chapter, but for now, I want to make the point that *anything* can be used *or* abused.

Consider sunshine, the source of all life on Earth. There is a vast and ever-growing body of science showing the numerous health benefits of vitamin D. More is being learned about this vital nutrient every day. The number of ways this essential nutrient interacts with the body in a positive way are too numerous to list here, but it affects everything from cardiovascular health and diabetes to asthma and calcium absorption. Some people say it could be the most underrated nutrient of all. That may be because it's free. No one's figured out how to charge you for sunshine yet, and that is the source of vitamin D. Sunshine interacts with a substance just below your skin and transforms it into vitamin D. Even only an hour or so of sunshine a *week* is sufficient to provide you with this life-enhancing nutrient.

That's why when I see people hiding from the sun because they've been convinced it causes cancer I want to scream. Yes, the sun can be abused by spending hour after hour in the sun, day in and day out; but by the same token, it can be judiciously used to reap the rewards it has to offer. Water can be abused also: if you dunk your head under water twice and bring it to the surface only once, you'll drown! Does that mean you shouldn't go near water, that you shouldn't drink water? You can use or abuse sunshine and water, and the same is true for proteins, fats, and carbohydrates. The sensible consumption of high-quality proteins, fats, and carbohydrates in the proper balance produces benefits for the body. It's the abuse of these three constituents of food, and by that I mean poor sources and overeating, that cause problems, and no amount of calorie counting is going to change that.

Creating a Calorie Deficit: Burn, Baby, Burn

To close out this chapter on calories, let's quickly look at what conventional wisdom states regarding their influence on weight gain and
weight loss. Simply put, a high-calorie diet is a fat-storing diet. Body
fat is essentially stored energy. If you are taking in more calories than
you are using up, you will not lose fat. To lose excess fat, you have to
figure out how to create what is called a *calorie deficit*. What exactly is
a calorie deficit? It is the process of burning or using up more calories
each day than you consume. The way you create this calorie deficit is
by either *decreasing* the number of calories you take in or *increasing*
the number of calories you burn off, or *both*. When you are calorie
deficient, your body is forced to tap into your stored fat reserves for
energy and the result is that you will lose weight.

Now all this sounds perfectly reasonable. But for me, I can't stand all
the keeping track. I said at the opening of this book that I love to eat, and
carrying around a pad and pen (or some electronic device) keeping notes
on every last thing I put into my mouth and essentially becoming a
human calculator around food does not appeal to me in the least. It takes
the fun out of eating and turns it into some kind of clinical endeavor.

And how would I even know how many calories I was burning up?
The body is *always* burning calories, even when sleeping! It's called the
basal metabolic rate (BMR), which is the total amount of energy
(calories) being burned or used up by the body while taking care of
internal activities like breathing, blood circulation, digestion of food—
that is, *every* metabolic process performed by the body. And that doesn't
even include the calories burned by physical activity! Interestingly, the
BMR accounts for the largest expenditure of calories, somewhere in
the neighborhood of 60 to 70 percent. How are you supposed to measure that? And certainly some people's BMR has to be faster or more
efficient than others are, so how would I know what range I was in and
how many calories I was actually burning?

Moreover, in calculating the number of calories I take in, how can I
be confident or assured that the numbers of calories I'm being provided

in each food are even accurate? Who says so? It's not as though there's some regulatory agency insuring that calories are measured accurately and that whatever is designated as in a given food reflects accurately what is actually in the food. Who really knows for sure? I'm just supposed to take someone's word for it and trust it is correct? And even if it is, I still don't know how to calculate accurately how many calories I'm burning. So, when all is said and done, not only am I supposed to do all this annoying, time-consuming calculating in and calculating out, I really can't be certain of how accurate it all is. It's *far* from a precise science. For me it's just not worth the aggravation.

Perhaps the most recognizable weight-loss program in the world is Weight Watchers, well known for its reliance on calorie counting. The now famous "points" system, which instructs dieters to lose weight by eating whatever foods they wish so long as portions are kept small, was revamped in early 2011. The president of Weight Watchers, David Kirchoff, had this to say about calorie counting on the Weight Watchers website: "The issue is that calorie-counting has become unhelpful. When we have a 100-calorie apple in one hand and a 100-calorie pack of cookies in the other, and we view them as being 'the same' because the calories are the same, it says everything that needs to be said about the limitations of just using calories in guiding food choices."

Calorie-counting has become unhelpful! That's putting it mildly I'd say. Seriously, do you know how overwhelming the evidence had to be against the concept of calorie counting for Weight Watchers to make such a statement, when the foundation stone of their success has been associated with counting calories for nearly fifty years?

Don't get me wrong, if calorie counting is something you want to undertake, fine and dandy. I'm not going to try to talk you out of it, but please reserve your decision on the matter until you have finished reading this book and have begun to implement the advice. Because between the Slender GR™ you will be taking and the dietary guidelines you will be following, you are going to be losing fat. And you won't have to take anyone's word for it either. You'll see the results on your scale and in your mirror.

2

THE GRANDEST GIFT
ENZYMES FOR LIFE

W HAT DO *YOU* THINK IS THE GRANDEST GIFT? What is more valuable, by far, than anything in all of existence? Frequently when that question is asked of people out of the blue, they quickly, kind of automatically respond, "What?" You know how sometimes when someone asks you a question that you absolutely heard, but you just automatically ask "What?" to sort of get your bearings and give yourself a brief few seconds to formulate an answer? Well, that's what usually occurs. Try it on people, you'll see what I mean. When I ask people that question, they usually think I'm seeking some esoteric, high-minded answer. Some think for a moment and say, "Love. It has to be love—to be so immersed in love that you love yourself completely and are able to love all others and are loved by others in return."

Others say the grandest gift is health—to be in a state of uninterrupted, pain-free, disease-free health throughout their lives, and for the same to be true for their loved ones. Still others say it's money—to have so much money that they and those they care for will want for nothing.

But back to you. What do *you* think is the grandest gift of all? Wouldn't you say, after serious contemplation, that it's existence itself—life—to be alive! For without life there is no experience of love, or health, or wealth, or anything for that matter. Life has been

31

celebrated in art, books, poetry, and music throughout history as the supreme gift, the ultimate gift, the grandest gift of all.

LIFE! YOU HAVE TO LOVE IT!

Consider the immeasurable vastness of the universe in which we live. It is indeed a daunting challenge to try to comprehend the impossible enormity of our universe. Our Sun is only one of *billions* of stars in our Milky Way galaxy alone, and there are billions upon billions of galaxies! Consider the astronomical number of factors that must have had to come together in just the right way and at just the right time merely to bring into being an atmosphere that would even support life. Then add to that the intricate and complex series of variables, raw materials, and occurrences that had to take place and come together with incomprehensible precision and timing to create life in defiance of all probability, and we can begin to see how rare and improbable our existence is in the grand scheme of things. We exist in spite of incalculable odds.

Richard Dawkins, in his book *Climbing Mount Improbable*, put it this way:

> So the sort of lucky event we are looking at could be so wildly improbable that the chances of its happening, somewhere in the universe, could be as low as one in a billion billion billion in any one year. If it did happen on only one planet, anywhere in the universe, that planet has to be our planet—because here we are talking about it.

I once read something on the improbability of human life, which I will paraphrase here. Picture one of those round, doughnut-shaped life preservers floating somewhere out in the vastness of the ocean being tossed about by wind and waves. Now picture a blind turtle swimming deep in the ocean waters. He pops his head above the surface of the water only once a year. Imagine if you will, the overwhelmingly implausible chances of that turtle poking his head out of the water in just the right spot out of millions of square miles of ocean, at just the right moment, to put his head through the hole in the life preserver. That will give you a hint of the extraordinary odds to which I am referring when it comes to the creation of human life. You know what? You're special! We all are! To say that planet Earth and her inhabitants are special might very well be the greatest understatement ever uttered.

Certainly you have marveled, as have I, at some of the astonishing photos from outer space taken by the Hubble telescope. The Hubble can take pictures, with remarkable clarity, of heavenly bodies that are literally trillions upon trillions of miles from Earth—distances so far they really can't fully be grasped.

Anyone who has ever gazed up at the heavens on a clear, dark night and marveled in wonderment at the vastness and enormity of the cosmos has probably asked this time-honored question of themselves: "I wonder how far 'far' is?" About 400 years after the first telescope was developed, the modern-day Hubble telescope was launched, and the answer to "how far is 'far'" has seemed a bit more reachable. Although the question will likely never be answered definitively, since infinity cannot be measured, the Hubble has nonetheless been successful in revealing to us the truly staggering immensity of the universe in which we live.

To begin to understand, even minimally, the truly astounding magnitude of the boundlessness of space, you must have a clear understanding of the term *light year*. A light year is a way of measuring distance. That may not make much sense because "light year" contains the word "year," which is normally a unit of time. Nevertheless, light years measure distance. Light travels at 186,000 miles per second, so a light *year* is the distance that light can travel in a year, which is just less than six *trillion* miles.

We toss around the words million and billion with such regularity that we tend to lose sight of the enormous difference between the two. In order to put them into proper perspective, consider that a million seconds is 11½ days, whereas a *billion* seconds is over 32 *years*! And a trillion is greater than a billion to the same degree that a billion is to a million. To further impress upon you how great a distance a single light year is, let us think of the space shuttle. The space shuttle is the fastest vehicle yet to be built, and it travels at 17,500 miles per hour. Now, even though it's difficult in the extreme to try and have a sense of just how fast that is, consider this: it would take the space shuttle traveling 17,500 miles an hour over *37,000* years to go a *single* light year!

Did you know that the very closest star to our sun is over 24 trillion miles away? In fact, when you look into the night sky and see the uncountable number of stars that appear to be in such close proximity to each other, that vision is only an optical illusion. In fact, all the stars you see in such prodigious numbers are all millions upon millions of miles from one another. And that's just looking at the stars in our Milky Way galaxy and not the *billions* of other galaxies separated by distances that dwarf the size of the galaxies themselves. Mind-boggling.

And yet, do you know what thing is most glaringly absent from Hubble's celestial travels and picture taking? Life! Pictures have been taken in every direction out into the boundless expanse and not a single blade of grass has yet to be detected. It appears that there is more life right here on our little blue planet than in the entire known universe combined. Could you even imagine the excitement that would be generated if something—anything—living *were* to be found out there? I'll bet it would be the lead story on the evening news every night for quite a while.

Whereas life is a rarity in the far reaches of space, here on Earth there is so much life I don't think we can help but take it for granted. The planet is literally bursting and teeming with life—absolutely everywhere. The profusion and diversity of life that abounds is staggering. Even in the most remote regions of all, where it can be so hot it melts you skin or so cold it freezes your blood, there is life to be found. How indescribably fortunate we all are to be here. The gift that is life is truly beyond description. Yes, life stands all on its own as it reigns supreme—it is surely the grandest gift.

Life = Enzymes = Life!

There are actually two ways of spelling the word "life"; the first is the traditional spelling, l-i-f-e, the second is e-n-z-y-m-e. Yes, all that stuff about the cosmos and planet Earth and the unlikelihood of being alive was all to introduce you to the subject of enzymes. And when the full measure of the importance of enzymes in relationship to all of life is taken into account, that description, and more, is totally warranted.

More and more of late, enzymes are being researched and talked about, and with good reason. Perhaps you have been hearing about them yourself but aren't quite sure exactly what they are or, more important, what an immense role they play in our lives.

You can describe an enzyme as a biological catalyst or as a tiny chemical protein—and both descriptions would be correct. But first and foremost, enzymes are all about life and living on this planet. Frankly, considering the unparalleled importance and incomparable role of enzymes in sustaining all life on our planet, I'm rather amazed that more people don't have a greater understanding of what they are and what they do.

When you look around at the astounding diversity of life on earth, in all of its glorious magnificence, it's interesting to contemplate the fact that none of it—not one scrap of it—would exist except for the presence of enzymes. Not one plant, not one animal, not one human being would exist if not for enzymes. Let me be very clear here, because this is not an exaggeration of the facts: Were it not for enzymes, planet Earth would resemble the other planets in our solar system that are devoid of life. It would be as barren as the moon.

My own introduction to the vital role enzymes play in our very existence came about when I first started my studies of diet, health, and nutrition in 1970. But it wasn't until 1995 that I learned there were totally pure and natural enzyme products available on the market that could assist the body in achieving that high level of health to which we all aspire. That is the beauty of enzyme therapy: it's not that enzyme products in and of themselves can heal physical ailments, it's that they actually strengthen, support, and assist the living body's own intrinsic effort to cleanse, repair, and heal.

As I discussed in the Introduction, when a word ends in "ase" it refers to some type of enzyme. Regarding diet, food, and nutrition, there are three basic categories of enzymes, each of which play a specific role metabolically and digestively:

❑ Protease, which breaks down proteins,

❑ Lipase, which breaks down fats, and

❑ Amylase, which breaks down carbohydrates

Note that within these three categories, there are actually *thousands* of enzymes. Scientists have identified over 5,000 enzymes that our bodies manufacture and utilize. In actual fact, there may well be tens of thousands of different enzymes within the body. Regardless of how many there are, each is a form of either protease, lipase, or amylase.

When protease, lipase, and amylase are being utilized to perform their respective functions in the digestive tract, they are called *digestive enzymes*. When they perform their tasks anywhere else in the body other than the digestive tract—for example, in body tissue, the bloodstream, and so forth—they are referred to as *metabolic enzymes*. Metabolic enzymes are defined as any enzyme produced within the body that is *not* utilized for digestion.

WHERE DO ENZYMES COME FROM?

We know we must eat food in order to obtain the nutrients and energy we need to stay alive. But the entire spectrum of nutrients carried into the body in food must in effect be "unlocked" from the food. And the key to the lock is enzymes; without them, nutrients would not be available to the body. Enzymes are the catalysts that make the extraction and utilization of nutrients possible.

Fact: You Will Eat Seventy Tons of Food in Your Lifetime!

Here's something that will likely make you raise your eyebrows in stunned amazement. On average, each one of us will consume somewhere in the neighborhood of seventy tons of food in our lifetimes. That's seventy tons! And a few of us are making a concerted effort to go beyond even that impressive total. But seventy tons is the average. When you contemplate the fact that seventy tons of food will pass through your body, it's not too difficult to see that even if the tiniest percentage of it is left sticking around in your body it will cause you to be overweight. Clearly, it's pretty much impossible to overstate the importance of having a digestive system that functions at an extremely efficient level. And it would seem to go without saying that one's enzymatic activity would have to be exceptional.

Where do enzymes come from? Well, unlike nutrients, which are transported into the body in food, enzymes are *not* acquired from food. Enzymes, in sufficient numbers, are simply far too crucial to the body's survival for their existence to be left up to chance or to proper diet. Therefore, out of necessity, enzymes are produced in the body. All living cells produce metabolic enzymes, although the pancreas, liver, and gallbladder play a vital, expanded role in determining and regulating the amount of metabolic enzymes the body produces. The enzymes produced continue working until they wear out—or, essentially, run out of energy. Once an enzyme no longer contains any energy, it will cease being a catalyst and will be treated like any other protein—that is, it will be digested and assimilated as a protein source for the body. (Remember what we discussed earlier: enzymes are defined as both catalysts *and* tiny chemical proteins.)

ENERGY, ENZYMES, AND THE HUMAN BODY

The living human body is an energy-processing factory, and an awesomely efficient one at that! It won't come as a revelation to anyone that energy is at the very essence of every activity of the living body. Energy is the indispensable commodity that makes everything you do possible and that makes everything your *inner* body does possible. People always want more energy. I've never heard people complain about the fact that they just have too darn much energy! But I've heard the opposite innumerable times. How about you? Do you have all the energy you need throughout the day or do you ever find yourself lacking?

I've mentioned that the living body has 100 trillion cells. And

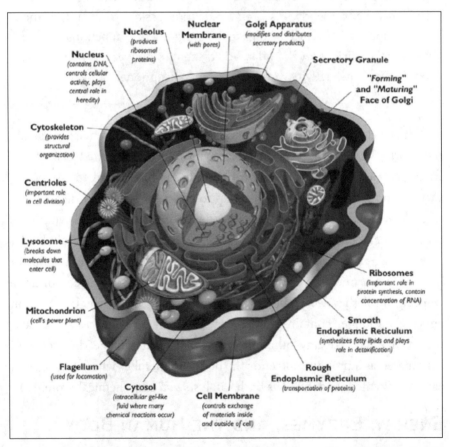

Figure 2.1. It wasn't until the electron microscope was invented that an individual cell could even be viewed to reveal its intricate and extensive workings. Each cell looks something like this.

every cell is a dynamically functioning miniature of the body itself. If you would like to do something that will really blow your mind, get your hands on a comprehensive physiology book, or go online, and look up renderings of what *one* human cell looks like. If you have never done this before you are in for quite a surprise.

It's astounding what goes on in each cell twenty-four hours a day. Each cell is bursting with life, bustling with unimaginable activity. Just as our body takes in food, extracts the nutrients and energy it needs from the food, assimilates nutrients and energy to carry out all the functions of life, and eliminates the residue, each of the body's 100 trillion cells are doing the *exact same thing*, performing millions of functions every moment. Actually, I'm surprised our bodies don't give off a perpetual, low-grade humming sound. And this is all possible because of energy.

Here's another rather astounding little physiological tidbit for you to ponder. Guess what activity of the body uses more energy than any other? Digestion! Have you ever felt tired after eating a big meal? That's like asking if you've ever seen the sun! Who hasn't? And you know, the bigger the meal the more tired you are. It's no accident that all over the world there's a little something called "the afternoon siesta." People eat and then they either have to take a nap or start consuming drinks with artificial stimulants just so they don't fall asleep at their desks.

In fact, and this is the really impressive part, not only does digestion require more energy than any other activity of the body, it requires more energy than *all* other activities of the body combined! There are some estimates that put the expenditure of energy for digestion at up to 80 percent. That leaves only 20 percent of energy reserves for every one of the other activities of the body necessary to perpetuate life— circulation, elimination, mobility, respiration—everything! Food in the stomach is a number-one priority as far as the living body is concerned. No matter what else is going on, no matter what else the body has to do, the moment food enters the stomach, whatever energy is necessary to deal with it is diverted to digestion regardless if it short-changes other activities and their energy needs.

Think of it this way: Imagine you have a bank account into which a set amount of money is deposited for you and your family to live on each month. What if your mortgage or rent payment takes 80 percent of that money? That leaves you only 20 percent to pay for food, car loan, gasoline, auto insurance, water and power, health premiums, clothing, school supplies for the kids, cell phone, computer, kitchen and household supplies, movies, eating out, vacation—*everything*! Now, imagine that your mortgage or rent payment *dropped* 20 percent. All of a sudden you have 40 percent to spend on everything else—*double* the amount you were making do on before. Do you think you would like that? I might as well be asking if you would like the car of your choice free of charge.

What I am trying to say here is that there is a way for you to use less energy for digestion and free up more energy for the other activities of the body, including weight loss. If you wish to keep your weight in check, and keep your overall health in good stead, you need to free up as much digestive energy as you can spare. Most people give little if any thought to the connection between their digestion and gaining or losing weight, but the two happen to be inextricably intertwined.

I'll share with you two means by which you can help your digestive tract use less energy in the process of digestion—and thereby create more energy to burn fat. Let me talk about one of those methods now, and the other one later in the book (see Chapter 4).

METABOLIC ENZYMES: YOUR BODY'S LIFE FORCE

The first way you can free up energy for fat burning is through—you guessed it—enzymes. Slender GR™, the enzyme formulation introduced in this book, specifically helps remove excess fat stored in the body. And, as it happens, there are other enzymes, equally pure and effective, designed to streamline the digestive process so that it not only functions more efficiently but it does so on *less* energy. To explain how this works, I need to return to the topic of metabolic enzymes, digestive enzymes, *and* food enzymes. (For more on Slender GR™ specifically, see the Appendix.)

Metabolic enzymes are referred to as the body's "labor force," and with good reason. The description of a labor force could not be more appropriate. That is because the literally trillions of activities that take place in the body every moment that allow life to unfold and continue uninterrupted, are entirely dependent upon metabolic enzymes. Without them life would come to a halt. If you were somehow deprived of the actions of these powerful little dynamos working tirelessly in your behalf, you would not be able to walk, talk, lift your arm, swallow food, or turn that food into blood, muscle, and bone. Your blood would not circulate, you could not breathe, wastes could not be broken down and removed, and cells could not be replaced. Not *one* bodily process, inside or outside, would be performed.

The point has been made that in terms of staying alive the body must be able to extract the nutrients and energy it needs from food. Even if you consume the most pristine, nutrient-rich, and energy-packed foods available anywhere in the world—ones bursting with every constituent necessary for the body to be successful in its efforts—they will all go to waste if there are not sufficient metabolic enzymes on hand to extract and utilize them appropriately.

Here's an analogy that makes this point well. Imagine a bridge that needs to be built over a body of water to connect one piece of land to another. You have all the materials you need to build a top-notch bridge: steel, concrete, wiring, mortar, cables, cranes, girders, and beams. And you bring all those materials down to the water's edge so they're available for the construction. But guess what? If there isn't a team of construction workers and an engineer to oversee them, no bridge will ever be built. All the components will not somehow magically assemble themselves into a bridge.

Metabolic enzymes are your body's engineer and construction workers, and without them there is *no* possibility of the living body benefiting from the presence of nutrients and energy sources, no matter the quantity or the quality.

Perhaps the most important factor associated with the production and availability of metabolic enzymes is the fact that only a finite number of them can be produced by your body. This is no small matter. In fact, it's a huge concern. I wish it were otherwise, but it is a physiological fact of life that the living body can manufacture only a certain number of metabolic enzymes and no more; when that limit is reached, that's it! You, me, everyone will eventually run out of metabolic enzymes; it's the natural design of the human body. And when that happens—well, there's no other way of putting it, but no more metabolic enzymes means no more life. Yes, the life of the body comes to an end.

Now before you start freaking out over what I'm saying here, I want to be very clear that this may happen when you are well into your hundreds. But as we all know very well, our lives will come to an end at some point. It's just that when that day does arrive it will be because the body's capacity to produce more metabolic enzymes ran its course. Imagine a bank account set up in your name at the time of your birth. Into that account a certain set amount of money is deposited, and it's designed to last your lifetime. Money can *only* be withdrawn, not deposited. Don't you think it would be wise and prudent not to squander that money haphazardly in order to make it last as long as possible? Yeah, me too.

Well, in the simplest terms, when it comes to metabolic enzymes, you have a metabolic bank account just like the one described above. Throughout the course of your life you will be making regular withdrawals, but you can never make any deposits. What you *can* do is see to it that there is no unnecessary squandering of your precious metabolic enzymes. This is something that is very definitely in your control. The greater the demand on your metabolic enzyme storehouse, the shorter will be the length of your life. On the other hand, lowering the requirement for metabolic enzymes results in a longer life. This isn't something that is negotiable; it is a law of life that is as intractable as the law of gravity. This next sentence falls into the category of, "Gee, you don't say?" In terms of your health and longevity, therefore, any measures you undertake that result in fewer demands being made on your body's metabolic enzyme storehouse are clearly the most sensible and intelligent things you will ever do—that is, if it is your desire to live a long time.

FOOD ENZYMES + DIGESTIVE ENZYMES: YOUR BODY'S WORKFORCE

What if I were to tell you that you can make your metabolic enzymes last longer and the means to do so is tied into . . . well, what do you know—digestion! I've told you about metabolic enzymes and I've told you about digestive enzymes. Now I need to take a moment and tell you about food enzymes. Do you recall me pointing out that all plant life, animal life, and human life is dependent on enzymes? As a fundamental part of nature's grand plan for life on earth, *all* food grown from the ground contains within it the naturally occurring enzymes needed for that food to be digested once it enters your body.

Here's the rub: heat destroys enzymes. It is a simple fact of life that most food eaten by most people is cooked. At 118°F, which is far less heat than is required to cook food, enzymes are destroyed. They are not merely damaged or weakened, making them less effective. No, they are, in no uncertain terms, obliterated. And we're not just talking about *some* of them; one and all are gone! As far as your living body is concerned, this is, to put it mildly, not a good situation. It is in fact a *bad* situation with some unwanted, destructive consequences. Remember, food cannot just sit there in the stomach waiting for the body to get around to initiating digestion. But because the food has been cooked, the enzymes that would have assisted the body with digestion no longer exist.

Here is how that works. When a fruit or vegetable is growing on the tree, plant, or vine, it is essentially attached to its life source; the naturally occurring enzymes it contains are involved in keeping it alive. Once it is removed from the plant and eaten, the same enzymes that kept it alive before it was harvested become digestive enzymes, and they wind up contributing to the digestion and metabolization of the food after it enters your body. In so doing, they take the burden of digestion off the body's digestive system.

In addition to the enzymes contained in food that help the digestive process, the body also contributes its own enzymes to assist in making nutrients available to the body. But significantly less enzymes are required when food is not cooked. When the food *is* cooked, its enzymes are destroyed and the digestive system is put in the unenviable position of being forced to produce *all* the enzymes necessary to digest the food. The body is forced to bear the *full* burden.

At that critical moment of being "overburdened"—which, quite frankly, the body perceives as an emergency—the awesome intelligence of the body I have been praising throughout this book kicks into action. And it does the only thing it can do under the circumstances of being shortchanged on the digestive enzymes it needs. It calls upon the mechanism in the body responsible for producing metabolic enzymes and forces it to produce, *on the spot,* the digestive enzymes necessary to digest the food.

Now remember, this is the very same mechanism that produces the metabolic enzymes that determine the length and quality of your life! And since there is only a finite amount that can be produced, in the most literal sense possible, every time you eat food that has been cooked, you are in effect inviting ill health and shortening your life.

I can hear some of you saying right now, "Oh, I get it. This is just your roundabout way of trying to convince me to eat only raw food— no thank you!" No, that is not my intent. Look, I enjoy eating cooked food as much as the next person, and I do so regularly. True, my diet consists of more uncooked food than cooked, but I am not going to try to convince you to stop eating all cooked food. But, I am as concerned about safeguarding my body's metabolic enzymes as I think you should be about your own. So I do wish to share with you what I have done personally to conserve my metabolic enzymes rather than squandering them unnecessarily on a regular basis.

I mentioned in the Introduction that Slender GR™ was not my first experience with enzymes. Owing to significant technological advancements that did not exist at the writing of *Fit For Life,* today "live plant enzymes" are now readily available in capsule form. When taken immediately prior to eating anything cooked, they perform the function of food enzymes that have been cooked away. They are of the finest purity and potency, grown and harvested in pristine surroundings without being compromised with heat or chemicals. They come in very small vegetable capsules, are totally nontoxic, and have no side effects other than increased health and longevity. Most important, they prevent the needless frittering away of the body's most valuable natural resource: metabolic enzymes.

I cannot fully express how grateful I am for these live plant enzymes and consider them one of the most significant and beneficial advances in the arena of health care in my lifetime. I half jokingly say to people that I have discovered the fountain of youth because, after all, they conserve metabolic enzymes, the determining factor in how long the living body is capable of performing the functions of life.

Sometimes in life we find something that just works for us, so it becomes a permanent part of our lifestyle. It could be the way we prepare a certain food, or the manner in which we interact with others, or the types of movies we like to watch, or certain products we are partial to, or the way we like to dress—it could be anything. That's how it is with me and taking live plant enzymes before eating anything cooked. Once I became fully aware of the extent to which they affect the length of time I will live, I started taking them in earnest whenever eating cooked food, and I always will. Honestly, I would just as soon forego eating than to eat something cooked without them; and for me, who loves to eat as much as I do, that's saying something.

A study published in the *Journal of the American Nutraceutical*

Association revealed that there is only a 2.5 percent chance of selecting a nutritional product in the marketplace that is both nontoxic and effective. So you have a 97.5 percent chance of selecting a nutritional product that is either toxic or doesn't work. But the company bringing these live plant enzymes to market is committed to seeing to it that any product they are associated with falls into that elite 2.5 percent category.

Everyone needs to make money; it's just a matter of how one goes about doing so. There is predatory money-making and there is compassionate money-making. The makers of live plant digestive enzymes and Slender GR™ personify the latter. Please don't miss the interview with Dr. Mamadou on enzymes in Chapter 7, which he so graciously contributed to this book.

3

· ·

CHOOSE LIFE

LIVING THE ADAGE
"YOU ARE WHAT YOU EAT"

P ICKING UP ON THE THEME OF THE previous chapter for just a
moment—life in all of its glorious magnificence: —Generally
speaking, can you think of a situation where death (or something
dead) is preferable to life (or something alive)? I believe you would
be hard-pressed to do so, since everything about this planet and our
bodies is all about life and living. I know it is incredibly fundamental,
even simplistic, to say it, but life perpetuates life, not death. How's
that for stating the obvious?

YES, YOU ARE WHAT YOU EAT

I want to turn now to one of my very favorite subjects—and at the
risk of stating the obvious once again, it is likely one of yours as
well—eating. No effort need be made to deny it—we're here to eat!
We're eating machines. We would have to be, wouldn't we, to be able
to plow through that seventy tons of food I mentioned in Chapter 2?
Think about it. Most of our internal organs are involved, one way or
another, in dealing with that seventy tons: either in the eating of the
food, or the extraction and assimilation of its nutrients, or the elimination of the waste it generates.

Except for when we are asleep, we eat about every four hours, and
even more frequently than that if you include snacks. Consider the

fact that from the time food is first chewed up and swallowed, until the waste from that food is expelled from the body, the entire process takes on average, three days. So really, there isn't ever a moment, day or night, that the body isn't working on some aspect of the digestive process.

Food plays such an integral role in our lives. "Dinner and a movie" is almost a way of life for some. Going out to eat with friends, meeting for lunch to discuss a business deal, or having a picnic in the park represent only a few of the ways food plays a central role in our social interactions. Sitting down to a celebratory meal is almost required at a birthday, anniversary, or wedding. Food is *such* a dominant feature of our lives that it is very easy to lose sight of the one most important and indispensable reason why we eat: to stay alive!

It's not as though we have a choice in the matter; we either eat or we perish. Food, right along with air and water, are the three indispensable requisites necessary for us to stay alive. Of course, there are disagreements galore within the dietary community regarding what foods should or should not be eaten, when to eat, how much to eat of each category and in what combination. Walk into a crowd and ask the first ten people you encounter what their opinion is on these questions and you're more likely to win money in Las Vegas than you are to find two of them to agree across the board. However, you can be assured that all ten of those people will unanimously agree that we must eat *something*.

There's a tired old cliché that I'm sure everyone has heard more times than they care to: "You are what you eat." Do you know what makes a cliché a cliché? It's something that is so indisputably true that there is never any disagreement from any quarter. Unless, of course, it comes from those who are so belligerent that they just like to argue for the sake of arguing. Without eating we will die—no doubt about that. Every day—in fact every moment of every day— our bodies are replacing old cells with new cells. Literally billions of cells in the body die off every day and are replaced at the impressive rate of around 200 million every minute! Guess what the building blocks are for those new cells? I can tell you they are not being built from good intentions; they are being built from the food taken into the body.

So, taking into consideration that we are, one and all, living beings on a living planet, and that we know, beyond dispute, that we *must* eat food in order to stay alive, and as stated so obviously above—that life perpetuates life, not death—what do you, as a rational, common-sense, thinking individual, surmise would be the most beneficial food to eat in order to stay alive and well: living food or dead food? No, it's not a trick question. This question is so elemental to life I practically feel embarrassed to ask it with a straight face. Could there be any doubt as to the answer? Could any lucid, logical, sensible person say with utmost candor that it would be better to eat dead food in order to stay alive than it would be to eat living food? And yet, guess which category of food, living or dead, dominates, by far, the diet of most people?

Dead Food versus Living Food

Years ago I use to counsel quite a few people one-on-one. Although I am not the type of person who likes to document everything I eat or suggest to others that they do so (unless it's something they wish to do), I did request that each person keep a meticulous record of *anything* eaten for three days prior to our counseling session.

Without fail, their lists revealed that they were eating approximately 10 to 15 percent living food and 85 to 90 percent dead food. I can tell you that I could have told them that without them listing everything—that's why they were in my office seeking help! Let me be brick-in-the-face blunt with you here. Forcing the body to exist on a diet so heavily dominated by dead food that it only contains a mere 10 or 15 percent living food is *asking* for problems in terms of maintaining good health or trying to keep one's weight in check. Not many people can do so, and for those who can, it stands as a most inspiring testimony to the living body's ability to survive and make do in spite of a diet almost completely devoid of life.

Living food is food that has not been cooked. Dead food is food that has been cooked. I've already explained how enzymes, the life element in food, are lost when subjected to heat and the extent to which it renders the food lifeless. Let us not forget about the other constituents of food as well. There are vitamins, minerals, phytonutrients, antioxidants, trace elements, and other constituents in food, some known and some unknown, all of which are important as well. Some of these constituents are very fragile, and the heat of cooking either destroys or seriously degrades them. What do you think would happen to you if you were submerged in water heated to 200°F? You would perish straight away is what would happen. It is no different for the delicate nutrients in food subjected to such intense heat.

Do you know that seeds recovered from ancient tombs 1,000 years old or more have sprouted when put into soil? However, even freshly harvested seeds of the highest quality, once heated, will not sprout. Why do you think that is? It is because once the life force in a seed, or any food for that matter, is subjected to heat, it dies. (See "Pottenger's Cats" on page 51 to learn about one of the most famous experiments conducted to show the benefits of living versus dead food.)

THE HUMAN ANIMAL

Everything on earth falls into one of three categories—animal, plant, or mineral. Since we are neither plant nor mineral, that leaves animal. We humans are in the animal category. We are classified as the "higher" animals whereas all the others are classified as the "lower" animals. We are considered smarter, more intelligent—in other words, superior. This is largely attributed to our more highly developed brain and our ability to think and reason so expansively. Not that the lower animals can't think and reason, they most certainly can, but not with the sophistication and aptitude attributed to us—the higher animals. At least that is the story from we humans who are quick to point out that *we* are "God's finest creation."

Pottenger's Cats

From 1932 to 1942, Dr. Francis Pottenger carried out a meticulous, thorough, ten-year experiment using 900 cats placed on controlled diets. Only two items of food, meat and milk, were used and were given either in their raw or cooked state. The results were so over-whelmingly conclusive and convincing that there can be no doubt whatsoever of living, uncooked food's superiority over cooked food. The cats fed only the raw food produced healthy kittens year after year. There was no ill health, no disease, and no premature death. Death came to those cats only as the natural consequence of old age. However, the cats fed on the same food, cooked, developed every one of humanity's modern ailments—heart disease, cancer, kidney and thyroid disease, pneumonia, paralysis, loss of teeth, arthritis, dif-ficulty in labor, diminished sexual interest, diarrhea, irritability so intense that the cats were dangerous to handle, liver impairment, and osteoporosis. The excrement from these cats was so toxic that weeds refused to grow in the soil fertilized with it, whereas weeds prolifer-ated in the stools from the cats fed the living, uncooked food.

Here is the clincher: The first generation of kittens born to the group of cats who were fed only cooked food was sick and abnormal. The second generation was often born diseased or dead. By the third generation the mothers were sterile. Dr. Pottenger conducted similar tests on white mice, and the results coincided exactly with those of the tests run on cats.

Oddly enough, it is our advanced brain power and expanded abil-ity to think and reason that also gets us into trouble when it comes to diet and health specifically—troubles that don't seem to affect the so-called lesser intelligent species of the animal kingdom. So it can be most instructive to study lower animals to see how we are measur-ing up in terms of our physical condition since we operate from superior thinking and reasoning and they operate more from instinct. To start, consider that we humans are the only species of animal on earth to cook all the life out of our food before it is eaten—*the only one. We* are unique in that regard. No animal anywhere in the natural world cooks it food. Their diet consists of *only* living food.

You might be thinking right now, *Well that's not true. A lion kills its food before eating it, as do other animals.* True enough, but they're not carving out a nice big filet and slapping it on the skillet either. Also, interestingly enough, when a lion takes down a zebra, wildebeest, or water buffalo, they eat these animals immediately. They are lapping up the blood and eating organs and flesh that are still alive with enzymes, nutrients, and other elements of nourishment.

What's more, have you ever noticed, perhaps on a National Geographic-type program, that when a lion or other predator takes down its prey, invariably it tears open the belly and eats the inner organs first, especially the stomach and intestines? Guess why? You see, carnivorous animals don't eat other carnivorous animals (except under extreme circumstances). Rather, they eat plant-eating animals. It's a physiological fact that we all need protein to live, lions included, and protein is built from amino acids. Plants can manufacture amino acids from air, soil, and water but animals cannot. They have to eat the plant directly for their amino acids or obtain them indirectly by eating an animal that has eaten the plant. That's why meat-eating animals instinctively eat animals that have eaten plants. And no matter what they eat, the plant or the animal, both are raw—no cooking.

Did you know that worldwide, over 25 million people die every year from heart disease and cancer alone? This does not include millions more deaths from other cardiovascular diseases like stroke, respiratory diseases like pneumonia, AIDS, diabetes, organ failure, complications from obesity, and various other illnesses. Animals in nature are *not* dying by the millions of these diseases. In fact, the long litany of afflictions that beset human beings does not affect animals.

"Uh oh, hold on there," I hear you saying. I know you're all ready to tell me about your dog or your friend's dog that is arthritic, overweight, diabetic, or has some other physical ailment. That's my point exactly! Animals kept as pets, or in zoos, or in some other way come under the influence of human beings, are the only animals to suffer the same illnesses as humans. What could possibly be more obvious? Left to their own devices, animals in nature, away from the influence of humans, don't get sick, let alone die by the millions.

There's no obesity epidemic, or even a weight problem for that matter in the animal kingdom; the *lower* animal kingdom that is. Animals living in nature do not become overweight. Not even a gorilla that appears to us to be overweight with their big bellies; that's just their natural shape. Putting on extra weight and trying to lose weight is something that is unique to humans. And do you know what else is unique to humans and nonexistent in the lower animal kingdom? *We cook most of our food before it's eaten!* I wonder if you're familiar with the comment, "Success leaves clues!" We should take a clue from our normal weight counterparts.

YOUR BODY'S GUARDIAN ANGEL

I can think of no more comforting concept than that of having a guardian angel. A guardian angel is described as an angel sent specifically to watch over and protect someone throughout his or her life. I don't know for certain if there are guardian angels, but the idea of them is surely a heartening one, wouldn't you agree? And there is no way I can complete this chapter without letting you know about your very own guardian angel for your overall health—and specifically your effort to lose weight. I usually group the two—health and weight loss—together as they are most assuredly inseparable. The way the living body works is that in a state of health, one is not overweight. I know there are people who say they are overweight but healthy. Strictly speaking, however, from the body's point of view, that's not really so. That's kind of like saying you're wet and dry at the same time.

Recall how I made the point in the Introduction that your greatest ally in anything you strive for regarding your well-being is your self-repairing, self-healing, and self-maintaining body. Remember: The living body's survival mechanism is at work 24/7, tirelessly making every possible effort to acquire and maintain the highest level of health achievable. And nothing short of death will cause the body to relax that effort even to the slightest degree until it fulfills its mission. As part of that never ending effort for optimum health and well-being, the body *knows* if there is extra weight being carried around and will do whatever needs to be done in order to remove it. All you have to do, in effect, is get out of its way and let it do what it does best.

This is where your body's guardian angel comes into play. You see, there are certain systems in your body that oversee specific tasks: cardiovascular system, digestive system, nervous system, respiratory system, reproductive system, and others. Each one has very definitive functions to perform and nothing else. One of those systems has the explicit task of keeping you alive and well by removing *anything* from the body that does not support overall health and well-being, and one example is excess fat. That system is your guardian angel. Its official name is the "lymphatic system," or lymph system for short. At this very instant, while you are reading this, your lymph system is hard at work on your behalf. To repeat what I said earlier, all you have to do is just get out of its way and give it free reign to do what it does best. You do that by giving it a fair share of living food to fuel its efforts.

Not that you have to become a "raw fooder" or eat mostly living food (not that I would ever discourage anyone from doing so). All you need to do is slightly increase the amount of living food you eat and proportionately decrease the cooked food you eat. Then you will see firsthand how capable and responsive your lymph system is in getting your body in order.

I know what an exciting prospect it is for you to find out there is something totally safe like Slender GR™ that you can take to help you lose weight, and we'll discuss it more later. I'm excited about it too, but for me, *this* is the most exciting part of this book: talking about the mechanism in the body charged with optimizing health and well-being. My own excitement stems from the fact that if not for the efforts of my lymph system, we would be talking about me in the past tense. I'll explain that statement in just a bit, but for now it is exceedingly important—and crucial to your success—that you understand that your lymph system knows you are overweight, wants to shed those extra pounds, and is fully capable of doing so.

Actually, I am amazed that a greater number of people aren't more familiar with the workings of the lymph system, especially in light of what a monumental role it plays in people's health and longevity. Even more bewildering is the discouraging fact that those people who *should* know all about the lymph system—health practitioners in all areas of the health community—know little if anything about how extensively involved it is in our very survival.

The Lymph Network: The Body's Garbage Collector

I doubt if there is anyone who has not heard the term *immune system*. We are constantly being cautioned about this or that negative effect on the immune system or admonished to strengthen our immune system in any way we can. You can no longer read or hear anything about the subject of health, diet, or drugs without the immune system being mentioned in some regard. Most people don't really know what the immune system actually is and couldn't give a very comprehensive description. Could you? When asked, most people just say something like, "Yeah, it's what keeps us from getting sick, right?" And even though that is absolutely correct, beyond that fact no one seems to know how it actually works and what can be done to strengthen, support, and optimize its efforts.

The heart and soul of what is commonly referred to as the immune system is the lymph system. It is a truly astounding network of glands, nodes, nodules, vessels, fluid, bone marrow, organs such as the spleen, appendix, and tonsils, and more. Miles of vessels contain *three times* more lymph fluid than the body contains blood. There are some nodes as big as a nickel, which you can feel on the side of your neck, under your arms, or where your leg meets your torso. There are others as small as the head on a pin.

You have likely heard the term *white blood cells* (leukocytes), which are antibodies the lymph system produces and sends out to scour the body, neutralizing and removing anything that does not support health and well-being. I cannot fully detail how unimaginably complex and extensive the lymph system is within the body. There quite literally is not a single spot *anywhere* inside the living body that does not come into direct contact with, or interact with, the lymph system.

What is it that makes it vital that every last cell in the body interacts with the lymph system? Perhaps sharing with you yet another name for the lymph system, other than guardian angel, will give you an idea. The lymph system is also referred to as the body's garbage collector. As you know, the living body is always involved in the process of metabolism. Food is being eaten and digested, nutrients and energy sources are being extracted and assimilated, and wastes are being degraded and eliminated. There is no time when one or the other of these activities is not being conducted.

As stated, every last one of the body's 100 trillion cells is carrying on all the processes of metabolism individually *all the time.* They are taking in nourishment, using what they need to fuel their innumerable activities, and eliminating the rest. Each cell in your body is producing its own amount of waste that *must* be collected and removed. And it is the final part of the process, the elimination of waste, that holds the key to your success in losing weight or in achieving *anything* in terms of your health.

There is no possibility of overstating the importance of eliminating wastes from your body. Uneliminated waste is the root cause of virtually every negative health issue associated with the living body, from overweight to serious disease and everything in between. If there was a way for me to make that last sentence blink on and off in red flashing lights so it jumped off the page at you I surely would. Since I can't do that I'm going to repeat it and set it off on its own in bold so you will hopefully give it the level of attention it most assuredly deserves.

There is no possibility of overstating the importance of eliminating wastes from your body—uneliminated waste is the root cause of virtually every negative health issue associated with the living body, from overweight to serious disease and everything in between.

Of course, there are circumstances when the body suffers due to other causes, like an accident, smoking, breathing in asbestos, or being poisoned by some type of environmental pollutant. But the vast majority of ailments that afflict people are caused by uneliminated wastes. Over the course of the last forty-plus years in which I have been studying this material, I have gathered a small handful of knowledge of which I am so certain, I would wage everything I own against a peanut that they are correct. And the importance of eliminating wastes in order to achieve good health is one of them.

You know what I find interesting? Whenever you hear someone discussing diet and health, the conversation routinely revolves around what should or should not be put *into* the body. I rarely, if ever, hear about what should come *out*. You ever notice that? Whether it's food or water or supplements, everything is about the wisdom of either putting or not putting something into the body. To be sure, it is wise to be prudent about what you consume regularly, but not to give equal importance to what is removed from the body is downright *un*wise. When you shift your focus and begin thinking more about the removal of wastes from your body, you will start to make the headway you desire in reaching your weight and health goals.

What are these "wastes" I am referring to? And more importantly, how are they generated? First, you should know the wastes I'm bringing to your attention are toxic—literally meaning poisonous—which is why they are referred to as *toxins*. Also, you should know that, strange as it may seem, they are a normal and natural part of existence, generated as a result of the processes of life unfolding. There will be toxins generated in everyone's body every day, and they will always be present to some degree no matter what. The healthiest people on the healthiest diets with the healthiest lifestyles will still have toxins in their body.

Think of the process of respiration—breathing. Every time you inhale you take in oxygen, and when you exhale you release carbon dioxide. There is no doubt that carbon dioxide is deadly, but it has to be present if you are breathing. The carbon dioxide is only deadly if it is forced to stay in the body.

It's the same with toxins; they're only harmful if forced to stay in the body.

There are two sources of these naturally occurring toxins, internal and external. Internal toxins are the result of spent (or dead) cells. Remember me pointing out that literally billions upon billions of cells die off every day in the body and are replaced with new ones? Well, those spent cells are toxic and would kill you if they just piled up every day and were not removed. The second source of toxins, the real mother lode in fact, is the consequence of metabolism. That's right, external toxins are generated from that famous seventy tons of food we eat in a lifetime.

Every day, throughout the entirety of your life, these two sources are churning out toxins, and it is the responsibility of each and every one of us to do whatever is in our power to support the lymph system's ongoing effort to get rid of them. Or be prepared to endure the consequences, which I can tell you ain't fun.

Fortunately for us, the supremely intelligent living body does not have to be forced or coaxed in any way into performing the vital task of waste removal; on the contrary, it is something the body initiates and undertakes for its own survival. It is as automatic as is the blinking of your eyes. You don't ever think, "Gee, I haven't blinked in five or six seconds. I better go ahead and blink now." Do you? Of course not, and in all likelihood you never would have even thought of your eyes blinking had I not brought it up. It is something automatic, programmed into the body's computer, for the lack of a better term. The body knows when the eyes need to blink and takes care of that for us without us having to think about it. And the same thing goes for the removal of toxins.

It is a physiological fact of life that the living body, as part of its very existence, is continuously generating wastes that *must* be removed or death will result. We know that an inexpressible intelligence governs everything about the living body down to the very last detail. Do you think there is even the slightest chance at all that this intelligence would somehow overlook something as monumentally important as providing the body with a means by which naturally occurring wastes could be removed? The mere thought of such an oversight is preposterous. It would be like building a billion-dollar aircraft and forgetting to attach wings!

The unwanted problems, including excess weight, associated with uneliminated wastes will only occur if more wastes are generated than are eliminated. There are two factors that can cause such a dilemma. The first has to do with energy availability. The lymph system operates on energy just like every other activity of the body. We know that digestion gobbles up the lion's share of energy, and no matter how much it needs, that energy is allocated to it, even if other systems, including the lymph system, have to be shortchanged.

The second factor that affects the balance of waste generation and elimination has to do with the lymph system itself. If a person's diet is such that the lymph system is regularly overburdened with toxins that need to be flushed from the body—or simply put, if it is regularly overworked—wastes are going to build up. When there is both insufficient energy *and* an overworked lymph system, well . . . that spells trouble. That's when all the mischief starts. Of course, under those circumstances excess weight will result; the wastes have to go *somewhere,* so they're "storehoused" so to speak. Where else will they go? They are stored in the tissues of the body until the lymph system is less burdened and has the energy available to get in there and move them out.

Here's an analogy that helps illustrate what I've been talking about. What do you think would happen if you never changed the oil in your car? Your car can be likened to the body in that you put in fuel, drive around, and as a result a certain amount of sludge is generated that winds up in the oil. Fortunately, all you have to do to rectify that situation is have the oil periodically changed and you're good to go—no harm is done. But if you don't change the oil, the car breaks down. With our bodies, we don't get to "change the oil." When sludge (waste) builds up in our bodies, we have to see to it that the lymph system's efforts are not hindered or otherwise thwarted from its appointed task of elimination.

If only people would show the same amount of attention to detail regarding the inside of their body as they do to the outside. When it comes right down to it, the outside of the body is just for show—the inside is what keeps us alive! I wish with all my heart that I could

How I Beat Agent Orange Poisoning

Let me share something personal with you that will not only make clear why I put so much stock in the power of the lymph system but will also illustrate what it can potentially do for you. In 1966, when I was twenty-one-years old, I was serving in the military and stationed in Vietnam. While there I was exposed to Agent Orange, a derivative of dioxin, considered to be the most poisonous human-made toxin in existence. As a result, I have a condition called peripheral neuropathy (PN), which severely affects certain muscles of the body, particularly the arms and legs.

Inexplicably, Agent Orange-induced PN can lay dormant in the body for ten to twenty years before any symptoms appear. In my own case, it was twenty years before a single symptom appeared—and that was in 1986. Usually, five years after the symptoms do appear (or what would be 1991 for me), those who are afflicted with PN are either in a wheelchair or dead.

Without going into a long litany of what this has meant for me, I will tell you that I limp significantly and have only very limited use of my arms and hands. As an example, I am unable to lift a glass of water to my mouth and can barely hold a pen to write my own name. However, even though PN can be fatal, and has been for so many others, I am fully describe the rewards in store for you when you take an interest in your own body's lymph system and do whatever you can to optimize its efforts. (For inspiration about taking care of your lymph system, see my personal story, "How I Beat Agent Orange Poisoning," below.)

KEEPING IT SIMPLE: FROM THE LYMPH SYSTEM TO DIET AND GOOD HEALTH

We are living at a time when the subject of diet and health has been made to appear so overwhelmingly complex and confusing that I

---

one of the longest known survivors to be walking around on my own without assistance.

I guess you have figured out where I'm going with this now. In 1970 (only four years after exposure and sixteen years before I would even know I was exposed), I was introduced to the importance of caring for my lymph system. It made so much sense to me at the time that I did whatever I could to strengthen and support my lymph system to deal with my weight problem and some other physical ailments I had, including what I referred to as "the stomachache from hell."

Not only was I successful in bringing my weight down and ending my stomach problems, but it turns out, my efforts to support my lymph system saved my life from the Agent Orange poisoning. I didn't know at the time that I had been exposed, but my body did! And apparently my lymph system was able to degrade the stuff at least to the degree that I had a fighting chance.

My reason for sharing this personal story with you should be glaringly obvious. If I could beat the odds and extend my life so dramatically against the effects of the most deadly human-made toxin ever concocted by strengthening *my* lymph system, imagine how much easier it would be for you to remove the normal, everyday, naturally occurring toxins in your body by strengthening *your* lymph system.

barely recognize it anymore. It isn't as perplexing as it is being por-
trayed. You are being misled! People have, for whatever reason, complicated the simple subject of diet all out of proportion to reality.
Exactly how could something so fundamental, normal, natural, and
necessary for life be so bewildering? How!? Seriously. Somebody tell
me—I want to know.

There is a virtual army of dietary advisors out there—doctors,
dieticians, nutritionists, naturopaths, the educated, the uneducated,
the serious students, and the dabblers—all vying to have their particular take on the subject heard and followed. Everything from good,
sound advice that can help you, to the other end of the spectrum of
utter nonsense that can harm you—and everything in between. I
guarantee that no matter what approach to diet resonates with you or
you adhere to, there is someone somewhere who will say it is the
completely wrong way to eat. Over the years, I have received hundreds of thousands of letters from people about this. And more and
more of late, I receive an increasing number of letters from people
who are simply exasperated and just say, "I am *so* confused!"

Hey listen, I know I am just one more of the voices out there and
the last thing I want to do is confuse you further. So I strive as best I
can to appeal to your common sense. I know there are those out
there quick to tell you what's wrong with your diet, who will advise
you not to trust your common sense because you can't trust it, and
you need to listen to them—the "expert." But I am convinced that
one's common sense is still the most reliable tool to lead you in the
right direction.

When I was first introduced to Natural Hygiene back in 1970 I
was sick and fat, and I was unhappy about it and eating anything that
couldn't outrun me. I *rarely* ate anything living. Never mind 10 to 15
percent living—I was eating less than 5 percent that was living. No
wonder I looked and felt like death warmed over. That's where I got
the idea of asking people who I counseled later on down the line, to
make a list of everything they ate. That's what was asked of me by
the person who introduced me to the world of healthy eating and

who became my mentor for years to follow. I'll never forget the look on his face when he first read over my food list—kind of a mixture of disgust and loathing. At first I thought I must have written something that insulted him in some way, and he was going to get up and punch me in the face.

No wonder it's so confusing out there; everything seems to contradict everything else:

❑ Eat lots of protein and very few carbs.

❑ No, eat lots of carbs and very little protein.

❑ Eat vegetarian.

❑ Eat macrobiotic.

❑ Eat all raw.

❑ Eat fat.

❑ No, don't eat fat.

❑ Count calories.

❑ No, don't count calories.

❑ Keep a list of everything you eat.

❑ Measure your portions precisely.

❑ Calculate exactly how many grams of everything enters your body.

Good grief! Do you *really* want to simplify things and guarantee a higher level of health for yourself? I'll tell you what to calculate. Calculate how much living food you eat each day—that's all you have to do. I'm not saying that to be flippant, I'm *serious*. You may not know it right now but living food is the key to your success in losing weight and keeping it off or in achieving any of your health goals. You don't have to keep track of a dozen things; you only have to keep track of *one* thing: am I supplying my body with enough living food?

Consider this, and please do so from the point of view of relying on your common sense to judge its worth: you know you are a living being on a living planet and you must eat to stay alive. Remember: life begets life! You must know that your living body requires—no, *needs*—living food. I'm not saying that you have to eat way more living food than cooked food (as great as that would be). What I am saying is that since it is glaringly obvious that more living food in your diet can only help you, why would you *not* want to increase the amount you are eating at present, especially if it would help in your quest to lose weight? Why would you want to knowingly deprive your living body of the one thing it needs more than any other in order to function optimally?

Considering the virtues of eating living food, does it not seem totally reasonable to you that *half* of what you eat should be living and half cooked? Does that seem *un*reasonable? Wouldn't that be fair—to your *body*? If it is true that the living body will excel on living food, does it make sense to deprive yourself of it on a regular basis? If you are presently eating 10 to 15 percent living food, or even if you are eating 25 to 30 percent, do you have any idea how bringing it closer to 50 percent would benefit your body and everything you are trying to achieve with your health and weight?

Over the years I have seen firsthand the results when people increase the overall amount of living food in their diet, and the transformation in their bodies that occurred upon doing so. Coupled with taking the Slender GR™ enzyme, more living food in your diet is a winning combination that can only bring you success.

I'm not saying that it has to be an overnight process either. It can be a gradual process that is comfortable and convenient for you so you enjoy the journey. As you start to experience results with more living food, you will naturally progress to more at your own rate. It's not a contest; you're not being graded. Do what is comfortable and doable for *you*. *Any* increase in living food will reap rewards and they will be noticeable, both in how you look and in how you feel. That's the best proof in the world. Don't believe me. Don't take my word for it. Try it and see how you feel. That's all.

How to Eat More Living Food: Salad Days!

Incorporating more living food into your diet is not a big deal. I can give you some easy tips. First, when speaking of living food, we are talking about raw, uncooked fruits and vegetables and their fresh (not pasteurized) juices, and salads, nuts, seeds, and sprouts. The easiest way to increase the overall consumption of living food in your diet is to make friends with salads. There's a lot more to salads than having a wedge of iceberg lettuce with a gob of mayo on it, which was my idea of salad before I learned better.

People who say salads are boring have never had one of *my* salads. There is no reason why salads can't be diverse, interesting, delicious, and satisfying. One reason why salads all too frequently have been treated with disdain is that they *are* often boring and unimaginative. That really is a shame because there are an endless number of creative variations for innovative and delectable salads. Not only can they be a tasty accompaniment to a meal, they can also be the central focus of a meal—which I'll explain in just a moment.

Let's just say, for the sake of argument, that you wish to get to that point of eating 50 percent living food and 50 percent cooked food, or at least closer to it than you are at present—even if that means a third or even a quarter of your diet is living. People generally do not think of a salad for breakfast; it's more of a lunch and/or dinner thing. What you want to do is look at your meal; is it almost all cooked with little or nothing living, or is there nearly as much living food as cooked? Obviously, upping the amount of living food with salad at lunch and dinner is a great way of approaching the 50/50 goal in a day's worth of eating. I'll be discussing breakfast in a subsequent chapter.

I know there are people who enjoy having their salad by itself, perhaps prior to eating the other part of their meal, and others enjoy eating it right along with the meal. Either is fine as long as it's eaten and not saved for the end of the meal—when you might be too full to eat the salad or wind up overeating just to say you had your salad.

I very much enjoy having salads either before *or* during a meal, but there is another way I like to eat salads that is my very favorite of all. Rather than the salad being eaten before or during the meal, it *is* the meal. This may or may not be a new concept for you, but it is fun, convenient, and enormously satisfying. And talk about endless variations. This was a concept introduced in the original *Fit For Life,* and I have been enjoying it ever since, as I am confident you will too. In fact, it may well revolutionize your notion of the obligatory or boring salad.

Honestly, what I am referring to here is nothing short of a major boon to enjoyably reaching your desired goal of increasing the amount of living food in your diet. These salads are easy to make, delicious, nutritious, and satisfying for both adults and kids. The idea is, instead of having a multicourse meal, you have a single course meal comprised of a basic salad with the other foods you desire mixed into it to make a wonderful, nourishing, multi-ingredient, gustatory delight.

Here's how it works: first you start with some basic salad ingredients, which can include lettuces, field greens, spinach, sprouts, tomato, cucumber, red cabbage, celery, carrot—you can have as many or as few ingredients as you like—there are no set rules. Then, say you feel like having steak and vegetables. Okay—you prepare the steak to your liking, cut it up in chunks, and add it to your salad ingredients. Then you can sauté up some sliced mushrooms and maybe onions, or steam some asparagus, broccoli, or whatever vegetables you like—and put them all in the salad. Add whatever dressing you are in the mood for, mix it up, and you are in for a treat. And it's 50 percent living food!

The same can be done with seafood—salmon chunks, shrimp, or some other type fish. Prepare the seafood you want, prepare some vegetables—maybe peas and asparagus—mix it together, add a dressing, and dive in!

Or maybe you feel like having a starch-type meal like pasta and vegetables. Prepare whichever pasta you like—penne, fusilli, maca-

roni, farfalle. Prepare the vegetables—again, choose what you like—
add the pasta and vegetables to the salad along with the dressing, and
there you go. Or instead of pasta and vegetables, perhaps you want
rice. Just substitute the rice for the pasta, prepare your vegetables in
the style you prefer, mix all with your salad, add the dressing, and you
have another delicious meal.

Maybe you just want to have the salad and vegetables. You can
prepare peas, corn, carrots, broccoli, cauliflower—literally any vegetables you like prepared in any way you like—add the dressing and
you're ready to go. Wow! Did I ever just make myself hungry!

I think you can see that the theme on these one-course meals
has limitless variations and is limited only by your imagination. They
are ideal for lunch or dinner and with a little ingenuity you could
have a different one every day for a year. I really hope you will try
these because I am confident they will be a welcome addition to your
eating lifestyle if you do. They are not only delicious, nutritious, life
enhancing, and easy to make, but they also significantly help meet
that goal of increasing your intake of living food in a most appetizing
and enjoyable fashion.

When eating these one-course salads, you may wonder if the
enzymes in the living food will also aid in the digestion of the cooked
food. The answer is no; living food only produces sufficient enzymes
to digest that specific food, not enough to aid in the digestion of the
cooked food eaten with it. Nor can they be stored in the body for
later use.

Snacking Your Way Through Living Foods

Another way of increasing the living food content of your diet is with
snacks. Everyone, it seems, likes to snack on something between
meals to "tide them over." But what you snack on can make a big difference to your well-being. I don't know why, but it seems like people
frequently have the attitude that because it's just a snack—a small
bite of something—that it really doesn't matter all that much what is

eaten. And they wind up eating something that is not very wholesome. But whether it is a full on meal, or a snack, it still fires up the same process of metabolism. Snacks can be a great opportunity to edge closer to that goal of approximately 50 percent living food.

I'm not only referring to carrot and celery pieces—which are fine, don't get me wrong—but other foods that can also be a tasty way of tiding you over between meals. Dried fruit is a good example. And there's a lot more than just raisins to choose from and which are also convenient and delicious. There is a very wide variety of fruits that have been naturally sun-dried or dehydrated without the use of chemicals such as sulfites. There are apples, apricots, cherries, mango, papaya, pineapple, plums (prunes), dates, figs, pears, and various berries. These are more concentrated than regular fruits and so stay with you longer to satisfy hunger, are a quickly utilizable source of energy, provide nutrients and fiber, and are delicious and convenient. Since they have their enzymes intact, they don't deplete the metabolic enzyme storehouse.

Now, some people may be apprehensive about eating such concentrated fruits because of concerns they may have about their blood sugar levels. I know this is a big issue for many people, and I will be discussing fruit and blood sugar issues specifically in another chapter.

Go Nuts!

Another equally beneficial snack is raw nuts and nut butters. Again, except for the sugar content, everything beneficial about dried fruit mentioned earlier is also true of raw nuts. I emphasize raw because roasted nuts are not that good for you. Everything good in nuts—and they are jam-packed with good stuff—is destroyed or deranged once roasted. They also are highly acidic in the body—not to mention the fact that they are dead due to the destruction of enzymes. But raw nuts are hard to beat in terms of something highly nutritious that really staves off hunger.

I am a huge fan of raw nuts and have them frequently. I'll share with you my favorite way of eating raw nuts. If you haven't eaten them in this manner it may sound a bit odd at first, but I hope you will trust me when I say it is *really* delicious. I eat raw pecans, walnuts, and pistachios with alfalfa sprouts, and raw cashews and almonds with cucumber slices or even celery. The flavor of these mixtures is truly something enjoyable. Also, raw nut butters on celery spears are another great snack. As I said, I hope you will trust me and try these snacks.

Both dried fruits and raw nuts are delicious, filling, nourishing, convenient, and help contribute significantly to the goal of increasing your intake of living foods. Both, as is the case with *all* living food, are also a good source of fiber, which most people know has numerous health benefits, not the least of which is it keeps one regular. And something else you can take my word on is the older you get the more meaning there is in that comment.

As I just mentioned, eating raw nuts with vegetables, such as cucumbers, celery, lettuce, sprouts, and so forth, works really well. They can be eaten alone of course, or even with fruit. Now, for some people, eating nuts with fruit does not work; it gives them stomach upset. But nuts are actually classified botanically as a fruit and work very well for many people. I like having nuts with grapes or raisins and even other fruits, which works well for me but not for everyone. Just experiment a little with various fruits and see if you are one of those for whom eating nuts with fruit works.

To paraphrase a quote from Edmund Burke, "There is no greater mistake in life than doing nothing because you could only do a little." Doing nothing will reap you exactly that—nothing! However, doing just a little bit, but on a regular basis, will ultimately turn into a lot! Consider this example of doing a little to gain a lot: If, after some natural disaster somewhere in the world, people were asked to send $1 to help the victims, one might think, *What difference is my $1 going to make in such a big tragedy?* But what if 100 million people from around the world sent $1? Do you think $100 million would make a difference?

The same can be applied to the effect of eating more living food on your quest to lose weight or generally improve your overall health. The beauty of adding living food to your diet is that every little bit helps. You don't have to eat all living food all the time or have only living food when snacking; you merely need to have the consciousness that however much living food you do eat will have a positive effect on your overall well-being. Take it slow. Don't let it become a source of stress or pressure in your life. Proceed at a pace that is right for *you.*

It simply doesn't matter at this point whether you increase the amount of living food in your diet by a great deal or only moderately. What is of greatest importance right now is that it be increased *somewhat*. Your body so craves living food that even the most modest increase will reap results. You will see what I mean. It will be strikingly apparent to you as your body rejoices in having more of what it needs to excel. Do a little, and it will turn out to be a lot! Just please don't do *nothing*. You do have a choice—I'm asking you to choose life!

For as long as I have been studying this subject I have been asked innumerable times what I thought about the four food-group approach to diet. Even a most cursory examination into the history of the federal government's excursion into giving Americans dietary recommendations reveals the undeniable influence exerted by business interests representing the food industry. Most influential has been the dairy industry despite *no* scientific evidence that a healthy diet *requires* dairy products. The first food guidelines issued by the USDA were published in 1916 and, oh, what a coincidence, that was only *one year* after the formation of the National Dairy Council!

Originally, there were twelve food groups. Then, in the forties, that was changed to the basic seven food groups, which was changed again in the sixties to the basic four food groups, then yet again in the nineties to the Food Pyramid and My Pyramid, which had six and five groups respectively, and again in 2011, to the My Plate Guide, which also has five food groups. All of these classifications have very little to do with promoting health and everything to do with not only keeping you confused, but also with big business feigning interest in your well-being in order to convince you to eat in such a way as to fill their coffers.

Allow me to simplify this subject: There are not twelve food groups, there are not seven, there are not six, five, or four food groups; there are *two:* living food and dead food. You want to lose weight? You want to feel better, have more energy, prevent disease, and live a long, *healthy* life? Eat more living food than dead food! There are those, I know, who will say that is far too simplistic an approach to health and well-being, but that is only because they have been as propagandized and conditioned as everyone else. Like I said, don't take my word for it; prove it for yourself. I can assure you of one thing: even the most outspoken, inflexible detractors of all would not suggest that eating more living food would *harm* you. What do you have to lose? Think about how you would feel if you discovered that I was right about what I am saying here.

For help in your living food journey, please be sure to check out some of the sensational living food recipes in Chapter 8.

4

Does This Go with That?

Combining Foods for Better Health

I WONDER IF YOU ARE FAMILIAR WITH the work of Dr. Robert S. Mendelsohn. Dr. Mendelsohn lived from 1926 to 1988. He was a world-renowned pediatrician and successful author, and it was my good fortune to be friends with him. He was a professor at Northwestern University Medical College and was at one time the darling of the medical community in the United States, so much so that he was made the Chairman of the Medical Licensing Board in Chicago, a most prestigious position for any medical doctor. He reached worldwide fame with the writing of his first book, *Confessions of a Medical Heretic*. It also ended his warm and fuzzy relationship with the medical community.

Dr. Bob, as I affectionately referred to him, was a man of impeccable integrity. When he could no longer live with the blatant inconsistencies and egregious shortcomings of standard medical treatment, he wrote his book to reveal all the failures and nasty little (and big) secrets of the medical profession for all the world to see. As you might imagine, the medical community was not the least bit pleased with his honesty. He was stripped of his chairmanship of the Medical Licensing Board, and his admiring colleagues, who had previously practically carried him around on their shoulders while heaping praise on him at every opportunity, turned on him like a pack of wolves.

A malicious campaign of lies and mistreatment was undertaken in order to discredit him and distance him from the medical community. Stories were fabricated that were designed to disgrace him and damage his reputation. One such story said that he had fallen and badly injured his head, damaging his brain to the point that his ability to think properly had been seriously compromised. The campaign didn't work. Dr. Bob's book resonated with people and he became a media sensation. He was an extremely kind, loving, and compassionate person and that came through in his interviews. People loved him. He wrote several more books, published an enormously well-received newsletter, and spent the remainder of his life in the limelight being praised for his work by most everyone—except those members of the medical community not enamored with his "lettin' the cat out of the bag."

Whenever he came to Los Angeles to do media, which was often, I always volunteered to drive him to all his appointments. He was so knowledgeable that I just liked being around him. One day I picked him up from the airport and on the trip to his hotel asked him how he dealt with his former colleagues turning on him and spreading such vicious lies about him. He looked over at me with his patented smile and said, "Harvey, always remember this—until you have been attacked by the powers that be, you can't really be sure you are doing anything of worth." I never did forget.

A few years later, *Fit For Life* was released and by that standard of Dr. Bob's, I was supremely confident that I was most definitely doing something of worth. Because the book so quickly became such a phenomenal smash hit with people, the "powers that be" of the day didn't take too kindly to some "uncredentialed" upstart revealing to people how they could improve their health and well-being in an area where the powers that be had failed. It wasn't that I didn't have credentials; it was that I didn't have *their* credentials.

No matter, I had to be discredited. The problem for them was that *Fit For Life* was not some radical approach to diet that required drastic nutritional upheaval. It didn't remove any food groups. It didn't require the consumption of special foods that had to be purchased regularly. It didn't fly in the face of common sense and reason, nor was it fanatical in any way. But they *had* to come up with something so they latched onto the one subject in the book that was most unfamiliar to them, that they hadn't studied, and that they didn't understand: proper food combining. And they went after me as though I were recommending that people become cannibals.

The thing is, no one could actually say that combining foods in a certain way was harmful, so the worst thing even the most vocal and outspoken detractors could say when pushed, was, "Well no, it's not going to hurt you, but there's no real science behind it." Of course that was not true, but whenever the "experts" are losing an argument, they quickly accuse those they disagree with of being unscientific.

Because of the popularity of *Fit For Life,* I was a frequent guest on every big talk show of the day. On one such show—I cannot recall which—I was pitted against someone there to discredit food combining. I remember asking him what books he had ever read about food combining or if he had read my book since he was there to lay out its shortcomings? His reply was something to the effect of, "I don't need to read anything about it. It's not rooted in science." When I pointed out that Webster's dictionary defined science as "knowledge attained through study," and that the subject of food combining had been studied for 100 years, he could not have been less interested. He was there to bad-mouth me and food combining, and whether he knew anything about the subject or not, by God, he was going to follow through on his mission.

My intention here is not to defend proper food combining—it proves itself too easily—but rather I wish to share the method with you in an extremely simple way and let you make up your own mind using common sense and logic. Do you recall earlier that I said I would share with you two means by which you can cause your digestive tract to use less energy in the process of digestion? The first is live-plant digestive enzymes; the other is proper food combining.

But first let me share my own story of discovering the benefits of combining foods.

MY HISTORY WITH FOOD COMBINING

I would like to share with you my experience with food combining to give you an idea of why I hold it in such high regard and why I want you to reap the rewards it has to offer. From the time I was a little tyke until I was twenty-five-years old, the most notable recollection of my life was the relentless, nearly unbearable stomachaches that plagued me every day of my life. I walked around doubled over most of the time trying to find some position that would give me relief for just a moment. All the doctors would say was that I had a "sensitive stomach," and so in a futile attempt to quell the pain I regularly swallowed an array of the most objectionable, vile-tasting concoctions—all to no avail. I gave up all hope of ever finding an answer to my predicament and just resigned myself to living in pain.

In 1970 I was introduced to the work of an extraordinary man named Dr. Herbert M. Shelton who lived from 1895 to 1985 and dedicated himself to the study of health specializing in digestion, which he studied for over sixty years. No one before or since has ever amassed such a vast body of knowledge on the subject of human digestion. No description could possibly describe the magnitude of this man's brilliance and dedication. He earned half a dozen PhDs along with several lesser degrees in various areas of the healing arts. He authored over forty books. For thirty-one years he wrote and published a monthly magazine. For over forty years he was the director of a health school and wellness center in San Antonio, Texas, where he personally supervised and monitored the diets of over 50,000 people.

When I first read one of Dr. Shelton's books on the subject of food combining, I couldn't help feeling as though he had written it specifically with me in mind. He explained that ill-combined foods could affect different people in different ways. For some, who are particularly sensitive, it can be disastrous. Not everyone suffers from stomach or other digestive pains, but those who do can be tormented by crippling pain for years and never learn the cause. They merely resign themselves to a life of agony. I remember thinking while reading what essentially was *my* story, *Man, oh man. I hope this has a good ending.* Did it ever!

My father died of cancer of the stomach in his midfifties, when I was only a teenager. He complained for *years* that his stomach was killing him. Little did he know! Now I'm not going to say proper food combining didn't sound odd to me, because it definitely did; it was contrary to the way I was raised to eat and had eaten my entire life. But the plain fact is, the prospect of being rescued from a life of misery, ending with cancer of the stomach, was such that if I found out that I had to combine crushed tree bark with lawn clippings I would have done so to end the suffering.

After reading the book I knew there was no way I wasn't going to try it. I mean, what if it actually worked? Plus, it was too darn easy not to give it a go. I never would have believed what happened next, had it not happened to me personally and only come secondhand from someone else.

It turns out I had *never, ever* eaten a single, properly combined meal in my life! I started to do so that very day, and in a matter of a couple of days, that was it—no pain. I ate and there was no pain. I couldn't believe it at first. The pain that had dogged me for decades was simply gone! And it didn't go away gradually over weeks; no, it was like someone showed up in my life, threw a switch, and bam! No more pain. I was dumbfounded. I kept waiting for it to return.

It's been over forty years and I've not had a stomachache since. I'm beginning to believe it works. And I'll tell you: when I hear some medical doctor, dietitian, or other type of nutritional advisor arrogantly dismiss food combining out of hand and declare it isn't scientific—or some other mindless, uneducated criticism as though they actually knew what they were talking about—I laugh out loud in their face, as do hundreds of thousands of other people who know better.

FOOD COMBINING: GOOD FOR YOUR TUMMY

The human digestive tract has some very definite limitations, and yet we have never learned how to eat in a way that respects those limitations. Those who insist on ignoring this fact are the ones who wind up overweight and ill. It astounds me that otherwise intelligent, educated people are laboring under the entirely unrealistic idea that they can eat any kind of food they want, in any condition (living or cooked), at any time (day or night), and in any combination, and as long as they can fit it into their mouth, chew it up, and swallow it, the body will handle it and everything will be fine. It is that kind of thinking that has contributed mightily to the obesity epidemic and less than stellar health statistics that dominate the population.

It simply is *not* true that the stomach is merely a bucket of some kind into which *anything* can be deposited for it all to slosh around together for a while before going on to be utilized by the body. All one has to do is look around to see the evidence of such a way of eating. Look around! Go to a mall or some other place where many people congregate and just look at them. Are they pictures of health—vital, active, and vibrant? Are they of a reasonable, manageable weight?

The living body incorporates an extremely sophisticated progression of highly organized and regulated chemical actions, interactions, and reactions. To deny this is to fly in the face of the most elemental physiological and biological principles that govern the living body. Some of these principles involve proper food combining.

The last thing I wish to do is to leave you with the impression that proper food combining is just too darn complicated to incorporate into your eating lifestyle. I know it can be made to appear so. I've read books on proper food combining that, had they been my first introduction to the subject, would have turned me off. I would have just said, "Hey, I'd rather be fat than deal with this." I'm into simple—simple and doable. So rather than risk turning you off to something that I *know* can help you, I'm going to give you the most uncomplicated, straightforward, and easy to understand explanation ever—the very basics of combining food.

The How of Food Combining

Other than fruit, which I will be covering in the next chapter, I want you to think of two food categories, simple and complex. Simple foods are plant foods—vegetables and salads. Complex foods are proteins (meat, fowl, fish, dairy, and eggs) and starches (bread, pasta, and all grains). The idea of proper food combining simply states that it is *best* not to combine a protein and a starch at the same meal but rather to have *either* a protein *or* a starch with vegetables and/or a salad. That's it! (P. S. Just a note regarding potatoes. Yes, they are a plant food, but they are so starchy they fall into the starch category.)

The Why of Food Combining

Now to the why of food combining. When you eat a starch, it can only be digested in an *alkaline* environment. Digestion begins in the mouth with a type of amylase enzyme in saliva called *ptyalin* and continues in the stomach with other alkaline secretions. When you eat a protein, it can only be digested in an *acid* environment. Foods are digested in the stomach largely by hydrochloric acid.

Have you ever taken an introductory chemistry course in school? I have a very vivid memory of a beginning chemistry class where a demonstration was given to illustrate perhaps the most basic of all chemical interactions. Into a large beaker of some bright red fluid, which was acid in its composition, was poured a small vial of an alkaline fluid. As they were stirred together, the bright red fluid *instantaneously* lost all of its color and the beaker was now filled with a completely clear fluid. It appeared almost magical to me as a young student. The demonstration was to show how quickly an alkaline and an acid in the same environment are neutralized. And that is exactly what happens to the alkaline and acid digestive juices in your stomach if you eat a starch and a protein at the same meal!

The consequences of digestive juices being neutralized in the stomach are not pretty; they are, in fact, nasty. In fact, as far as the body is concerned it is an emergency. Food cannot just sit around in the stomach. Not only does the metabolic enzyme mechanism have to be called upon to supply more digestive enzymes—an unfortunate waste of the body's precious resources—but more digestive juices also have to be secreted. However, upon the arrival of more digestive juices they are once again neutralized. Whereas food usually stays in the stomach for around three hours, it is now forced to be there far longer as the body struggles to do what needs to be done to finally move the food out of the stomach and into the intestines.

The problem with food hanging around for such a long time in the stomach is that the proteins putrefy and the starches ferment. It is, in no uncertain terms, a big, foul mess of rotting, putrid spoilage. Sorry. I know this description does not create a very pleasant image. But this is what many people put their bodies through three times a day every day of their life. No wonder there are so many sick and overweight people. Why do you think some people will throw up food eaten six, seven, even eight hours or more earlier? It's only supposed to be there about three hours. What's it still doing in the stomach eight hours later? It was *so* foul the body would not allow it to pass into the intestines, evidenced by its offensive odor once regurgitated. How do the food combining deniers account for this? They can't!

Do you know that every year one of the pharmaceutical industry's biggest selling categories of drugs are the ones prescribed for some type of stomach or digestive disorder? Consider some of these ailments: stomachaches, gas, bloating, heartburn, indigestion, acid reflux, constipation, irritable bowel syndrome, gastritis, colitis, Crohn's. Good grief! I'll ask the question I asked earlier: Why in the world, after doing something as normal, natural, and necessary to life as *eating*, do millions of people have to run straight to the medicine cabinet and barrage their bodies with drugs? For eating! You don't think there's something just a tad wrong in that scenario.

Now, I'm not saying that properly combining food will eliminate all of these digestive disorders. But literally tens of thousands, of the hundreds of thousands of people who have written me, have said specifically that combining their foods relieved them of painful stomach and intestinal problems that plagued them for *years*. Many said they were able to completely stop taking drugs, which never did anything to remove the cause anyway. All drugs did was fight the symptoms; the next meal brought the same discomfort. But after properly combining their foods, these people no longer needed drugs. What do you think these people would say to those who insist that properly combining food is a waste of time? Do you think their reaction might be, "Oh gee, well, in that case, I guess I'll go back to the way I was eating and stock back up on my Prilosec?" Yeah, right.

There are bound to be those who will point out that they ill-combine foods all the time and rarely suffer from stomach or digestive problems, I know—not everyone does. But everything is ultimately tied to digestion in some way. I would ask those same people how their energy level was. Lots of energy all the time? Do they ever get headaches, skin problems, or aches and pains anywhere else in the body? Sooner or later, incorrectly combining foods *all the time* is going to take its toll, and it just won't be attributed to what went on in their stomachs over the years.

Dr. Norman W. Walker was one of the most knowledgeable health practitioners the world has ever known. He authored several books and was recognized the world over as a preeminent student and teacher of health, which he studied his entire adult life. He lived an extremely healthy life and passed healthfully in his sleep at the age of 100 completely free of any physical ailments. This is what he had to say on the subject of proper food combining:

"These results are very real and not mere fantasy or theory. They have been proved far too often to leave any room for doubt in the mind of any but those who love their meat and potatoes so inordinately that they become blinded to the facts.

One thing in this life that I shall never understand is the fact that a chemist, of all people, whose intensive education is closely woven into an understanding of the effect of the combination of chemicals, would not dream of the incompatible mixtures in his laboratory, that he daily pours into his own body."

FOOD COMBINING AND STARCHES: A SPECIAL NOTE

One of the food categories I've been discussing warrants special attention here because it plays an overwhelming role both in greatly contributing to unwanted weight and in severely thwarting the body's efforts to remove excess weight. I'm talking about starches— that seemingly endless array of foods made from grains. In fact I would go so far as to say that if people did nothing but remove every trace of processed starch foods from their diet, not only would we not have an obesity epidemic but people being even moderately overweight would not be the problem it is.

Just to be sure you know exactly what I mean when I refer to processed starches, they include all breads, bagels, and so forth; pasta and noodles; cakes, cookies, doughnuts and other pastries; crackers, chips, and pretzels; all types of cereals, hot and cold; and rice and other edible grains. I think you get the picture—you know, all the "good stuff." It's so funny—well, not *funny*—but so many people are attracted to the very foods that are the worst for them. I know I am.

My personal opinion is that we humans are not natural grain eaters, biologically speaking. We eat them—oh, brothers and sisters, do we eat them—but they are not part of our *natural* inclination. There had to be a time in our collective ancient history that there were no starch foods like the ones I just listed. They came along with the advent of agriculture, which is approximately 10,000 years old. I don't know how far back the human species goes, but in 1994 some extremely sophisticated and remarkably well-preserved cave paintings were discovered in France. Carbon dating puts them at about 32,000 years ago, making them the oldest paintings of their kind ever uncovered. That's more than *three times* as long ago as agriculture.

One has to wonder what our ancestors were eating for those 20,000 years or so before we figured out how to grow grain and make foods from them. You can be sure there wasn't any macaroni, white bread, or doughnuts. Common sense would suggest that they were eating fruits, vegetables, nuts, seeds, and animal protein. What else was there?

But along came agriculture, and that was the beginning of the end in terms of the health of our species. Not right away, obviously. Ironically, for thousands of years people were using whole grains, which had *some* nutritional value. Until about 1880 in the United States, only stone-ground wheat was available. But along with the industrial revolution came what was called roller milling, which resulted in every vestige of life being lost from the grain to make flour in what was called the "refining process." This is where we get the term "refined flour." Oddly enough, physicians of the day actually condemned the practice. But, as is usually the case, economic and financial considerations won out.

Starches Are Harbingers of Death

Usually, when you think of the term "refined," it has a positive connotation. You think of someone who is elegant, educated, and well dressed, someone who has very polished social skills—someone who is "well-heeled." But when referring to flour that is refined, *nothing* positive is associated with it. Bluntly speaking, it becomes a harbinger of death, nothing more than a convenient and unfortunately pleasant-tasting delivery system for some of the most health-destroying substances you can put into your body: refined flour, refined sugar, refined salt, saturated fat, and an ocean of chemical additives.

Refined white bread is totally nutritionally deficient; anything of value naturally present in the grain used to make the flour is refined out. It's not just that it's worthless; if the body cannot efficiently rid itself of the residue, it is the type of carbohydrate that very quickly turns to fat. Did you know that in the early part of the twentieth century, darker, whole-grain bread was considered a sign of poverty by the "upper class"? Refined, worthless, white bread was actually sought out, not because it was superior nutritionally—clearly it was anything but—but because it was associated with one's class status. Boy, what a horrid example of "the joke's on you!"

Dr. Norman Walker, who I quoted earlier, was convinced beyond any possible doubt that starches do not have a single saving grace and eating them would have a more deleterious effect on one's health than any other dietary practice. He and I would have gotten along great.

Here's the big problem with eating starch foods. The small intestine is the organ in the body in which most digestion occurs. All along the intestines are millions of the tiniest little, fingerlike blood vessels called *villi* that protrude from the surface, absorb nutrients from food, and pass them into the bloodstream for delivery to the cells. The *only* way nutrients can be extracted and passed through the villi is if the food is first liquefied. No matter what you eat, it ultimately has to be liquefied before anything it contains can be utilized.

White Bread Banned as Fish Bait!

Here's a fun fact for you: In June 2011, a fishery in the United Kingdom banned anglers from using white bread for bait. Slices of white bread were routinely thrown into the water to entice the fish to come closer to the surface. Only thing is, the fish were eating it and becoming fat and lethargic! So now the use of white bread as bait has been banned. The comedian in me wants to run with this and do a routine about people eating white bread, but that would just be too easy.

That definitely makes sense when you consider that more than 70 percent of the human body is water. Here's the punch line—are you ready? *Starch is not water-soluble!* And that spells trouble.

Starches Spell T-r-o-u-b-l-e!

The fact that starch is not water-soluble is no small matter; on the contrary, it is a gigantic matter. Starch can't be dissolved and lique-fied so it remains a solid inside you and therefore cannot be utilized by the body. The undissolved starch molecules remain in the body and gum up the works as it were, clogging and interfering with blood flow, lymph flow, optimum function of organs, and efficient elimina-tion. The body gallantly strives to get rid of the stuff by storing some as—take a guess—fat! No diet will fatten someone up faster than a grain-based diet. Why do you think the big stockyards feed so much grain to their cattle? It's to fatten them up as quickly as possible. And it works!

Ever know anyone with kidney stones or gallstones? Not fun! How much would you like to bet that these people are fond of starches? In fact, when people ask me about how to deal with stones I start describing their heavy, starch-based diet to them, and they usu-ally say, "How'd you know that?"

Ever had any pimples or other blemishes on your skin? Bear in mind that not only is the skin the largest organ of the body, but it is also an eliminative organ along with the bowels, bladder, and lungs. One means by which the body rids the system of excess toxins that can't be handled by normal channels is to expel them directly through the millions of pores on the skin. Certain bacteria thrive more on starchy matter than on almost any other matter. As a result, they "help" us out by breaking down built-up starch molecules into pus, which is then pushed out through the skin—pimples!

Consider another fact. In the United States alone there are more than 2 million people who have celiac disease. These are people who cannot tolerate gluten, the protein component found in grains—most notably wheat, barley, and rye. These people are, in my opinion, the ones who are most sensitive to grains. I know their aversion is associated with gluten specifically, but the fact is, gluten or not, starch is not soluble in the body and therein is the root of the problem.

Look, I'm not trying to convince you never to eat starches again. I eat them myself. This all comes under the category of "know your enemy." Knowing what I do about starches, there are certain measures I take to mitigate the harm. First, I eat them minimally, and as often as I can, I properly combine them—meaning I don't have protein with starch. It's hard enough for the body to deal with starches all on their own; adding proteins to the mix and neutralizing the digestive juices is simply asking for grief. Instead, I have vegetables and/or a salad with starch foods, and *whenever* I eat starches, whether I eat them properly combined or not, I *always* take digestive enzymes. In this way at least I'm giving my body a fighting chance.

So, regarding properly combining your meals—and just to be sure you understand—if you wish to have some kind of animal protein (meat, fowl, fish, chicken, eggs), have it with a salad or vegetables or both. On the other hand, if you wish to have some kind of starch (bread, pasta, rice, and so forth), have it with a salad or vegetables or both. It is that simple. Remember our discussion about living foods in Chapter 3? When I described the one-course salads to you, I intentionally described them according to these same guidelines: they were either protein based or starch based.

Please be clear about something: I am not suggesting you have to combine your meals properly every time you eat. These guidelines are for you to use as often as it is convenient. We're talking about a lifestyle here, not a forced march. Sometimes you are going to want pizza, or a ham and cheese sandwich, or pasta with shrimp, or any number of other dishes that are not properly combined. Hey, come Thanksgiving I don't want to decide if I want turkey *or* stuffing—I want both! What is of far greater importance is the direction in which you are going, foodwise, not what you do at every single meal.

All I ask of you is that you try it. See how you feel when you properly combine proteins and starches and see how you feel when you don't. If you're home and it's convenient, fine. If you're out with friends, or at a luncheon, and you just want to have what's in front of you, fine. As I said, this is not a military exercise; it's a way of life. However much you can do will be beneficial. But remember: don't do nothing because you can only do a little.

What I will tell you is if you properly combine your foods on some regular basis, you will notice that you feel not quite as full or tired after eating; you will have more energy and feel less discomfort. And you will, as other people have reported, start combining foods properly more often because you will *want* to, not because someone is guilting you into it. That's when you know something is worthwhile and valuable in your life—when you are doing it because it makes you feel noticeably better, and because you have a genuine desire to do so. That, I am confident, is what awaits you when you start properly combining food.

5

IS THERE A PERFECT FOOD?
THE SWEETEST PRIZE

WHEN I FIRST SAT DOWN TO BEGIN writing this book, I was excited about introducing you to Slender GR™, the amazing new weight-loss enzyme. I was also looking forward to sharing the good news with you about your body's astounding lymph system and its ability to work tirelessly for you in your effort to reach your health goals. In fact, I was enthusiastic about the entire prospect of sharing the contents of this book with you. But I have to tell you, it was *this* chapter—Chapter 5—that I was most eager to write. The very instant I decided I would write the book, I started to think of this chapter and began jotting down notes about the specific areas I wanted to be absolutely sure I covered. After every other chapter I completed, I thought to myself, *Okay, I'm that much closer.*

You might be wondering what it is about this particular chapter that so motivated me. The answer is that it is all about my all-time favorite food this good earth has gifted to all her inhabitants. The one food, above all others, that when eaten *correctly* can do more than any other food to support the living body in its never-ending effort to acquire and maintain good health.

In case you haven't noticed, the theme of this book is all about life and living, not death and dying. The food to which I am referring, and which I will name in just a moment, is above all else a living food bursting with every element necessary to promote health and well-being. I am as certain of this as I am of the importance and necessity of eliminating wastes from your body for any real measure of long-term vibrant health to be enjoyed.

FRUIT! THE PERFECT FOOD!

There *is* a perfect food you can eat, and that food is fresh fruit! What was your *very first* emotional, not intellectual, reaction to seeing the word "fruit"? Was it one of revulsion that made you scrunch up your face in disgust and recoil as though I had described something revolting? Or are you actually a bit surprised that I would even use such words to describe a possible reaction to something that is pretty much universally viewed as, at the very least, a treat?

As someone who has studied this subject for over forty years, someone who has a special affinity for the nature of fruit, and who knows firsthand the extent to which fruit has been instrumental in my own health journey, I can tell you with a mixture of rock-solid certainty and deep-felt sadness that no other food has been more egregiously misunderstood or more unfairly maligned—much to the detriment of those who have been misled. The only thing that can account for this paradox is plain old, unmitigated ignorance. I don't use that word to be insulting or confrontational; I use it because there is no other word that can more aptly describe the situation. Being ignorant of something is not in and of itself a bad thing, it simply means a lack of knowledge on a given subject. Hey, I'm ignorant about many things; I have no problem acknowledging that. But the nature of fruit and its affect on human health isn't one of them!

When I hear some of the mind-numbing absurdities associated with fruit from people generally considered knowledgeable, I cannot help but be concerned for the people who are unjustly influenced. It brings to mind two famous quotes. The first is from George Bernard Shaw: "Beware of false knowledge; it is more dangerous than ignorance." The second is from Artemus Ward: "It's not so much what folks don't know that causes problems; it's what they do know that just ain't so."

This is precisely the challenge I face in bringing to your awareness the truth about nature's perfect food, which has been so unjustly cast in a negative light by people who know a whole lot about what is not so.

FRUITS ARE CARBOHYDRATES!

Contributing in a major way to the confusion that dominates this subject is the fact that fruit is in the carbohydrate classification. Proteins and fats are straightforward; there's not very much confusion over what they are and how they are utilized in the body. But the carbohydrate category—good grief! It's no wonder there is so much confusion and misinformation out there.

Proteins are essentially animal products. Fats are essentially oils and butter. But look at the carbohydrate category: all fruits and vegetables; all manufactured starch products made from refined grains, of which there are *hundreds;* and all manufactured sweet products made from refined sugar, of which there are also hundreds. In the *same* category, there are items that can assist the body in its life processes like fresh fruit and vegetables, and others like aspartame and high fructose corn syrup (HFCS) that haven't a single redeeming quality and can in fact destroy the body's health.

Because fructose is in fruit and also in HFCS, there are those who think that because of their chemical similarities they are actually treated similarly in the body. That's not just ignorance, that's ignorance squared! It would be like saying that all water is treated the same in the body. I guess, given that reasoning, since a glass of water from a clear mountain stream and a glass of water from the ocean are both chemically H_2O that would mean it wouldn't matter which one was consumed. Except for the fact that if you drink the stream water for a month it will be beneficial, and if you drink ocean water for a month it will *kill* you.

I will get to the subject of fructose in just a bit, but for now, I know that it would be easier than falling off a log to discuss this particular subject by burying you under an avalanche of physiological terminology, describing every step along the way that transpires from the time you eat a carbohydrate until it burns off as energy. But for what purpose? Bogging you down with the minutiae of a rather sophisticated, multifaceted process isn't really going to give you a better grasp of what takes place and *why*. And besides, whatever anyone thinks they know about the process is only part of the story of what the living body accomplishes; it's only what has been grasped thus far. No one really knows the full extent of exactly what the body is doing and how it does what it does. Yes, steps along the way can be described, but there are subtleties going on outside of our awareness on a level that we may never fully grasp. It's like trying to understand how the apple is turned into blood.

So I am going to stick with my approach of keeping it simple and not creating more confusion than already exists by loading you up with every little detail in the process of turning food into utilizable energy. It's like a lot of things that can be described either in simple or complicated fashion. It would be accurate to tell you that you must put gas in your car so when you press down on the gas pedal the car moves, and when you run out of gas you must refill the tank with more. Or I could tell you all about the internal combustion engine and when you press down on the gas pedal a mixture of air and fuel is drawn into the crankcase from the carburetor through an intake valve, which forces the movement of a piston up and down, creating pressure, then a spark plug creates a spark to ignite the gasoline, which produces a little explosion—resulting in the power to move the car. Catch my drift? I'll be using the simpler explanation.

Any understanding of the carbohydrate/sugar/energy dynamic *must* begin with what is considered the most sophisticated, awesome creation in all of existence: the human brain. In the Introduction, I touched upon the brain's ability to ceaselessly coordinate and direct the trillions of functions of the living body by orchestrating the activities of 100 trillion individual cells. Talk about not being able to grasp the highly developed intricacies of a mechanism outside the realm of our understanding! Granted, quite a bit is known about the brain, but the people who have made it their life's work to study this extraordinary organ say that what we know is dwarfed by what we don't know, and a full understanding may never be achieved.

FRUIT, GLUCOSE, AND YOUR BRAIN

Much disagreement abounds among people who discuss weight loss in relation to the optimum fuel necessary to drive both *that* effort and all of the body's other activities. But there also are some areas of total, unanimous agreement. For example, *nothing* within the living body gets done outside of the scope or jurisdiction of the brain, and the only way the brain can perform its assigned tasks is by being supplied with fuel on a regular basis.

Even the most obstinate contrarians acknowledge that the brain burns one fuel and one fuel only for energy. That fuel is glucose, a form of sugar. The brain cannot burn protein directly. It cannot burn fat directly. It cannot burn starch directly. No matter what enters the living body, it must first be turned into glucose or it cannot be used by the brain. This is no more open for debate than is the fact that the Earth is round not flat, or that the Sun is hot, not cold. The absolute, indisputable, physiological fact is that the brain can burn glucose and nothing else.

When we discussed calories earlier, the point was made that of the three categories of food we eat, it is carbohydrates that are responsible for providing fuel energy to power the living body. That process begins with the consumption of carbohydrates and the subsequent extraction of its sugars known as glucose. With the help of insulin, the bloodstream transports glucose to the cells as needed.

You have likely heard the term *low blood sugar* or what is also referred to as *hypoglycemia*. The brain is constantly monitoring the bloodstream to be certain there is sufficient glucose available so it is never shortchanged the glucose it needs to perform its multitude of functions. And should those glucose levels start to dip, the brain snaps into action and sees to it that the situation is brought to your

attention in no uncertain terms with strong and unmistakable warn-
ing signs: extreme hunger, trembling, weakness, nervousness, profuse
sweating, heart palpitations, even difficulty speaking.

This is not to imply that the brain has to wait around until more
carbohydrates are eaten to build up glucose in the blood. Until that
does happen, as part of the brain's ability to see to it that the well-
being of the body is not endangered because of insufficient glucose, it
takes steps to store glucose for just such an occasion. Glucose is not
only found in the blood, it is also stored in muscle cells and the liver.
Stored glucose is called *glycogen*.

The liver is referred to as the body's "laboratory" because, believe it
or not, it has well over *500* functions and is tied to every bodily
process. It is still uncertain exactly how many functions the liver per-
forms. Frankly, as is the case with the brain, no one really knows the
full extent of the liver's activities. But one thing is for sure: it's the
most important storage system for processed glucose in the form of
glycogen. So the liver not only regulates the level of glucose in the
blood, but in order to restore balance, it also releases glycogen in the
form of glucose as needed by the body for energy.

I've certainly not been shy in my praise of the incomprehensibly
intelligent living body, and the longer one studies it the more impressive are the seemingly endless, highly sophisticated mechanisms
designed to insure its own survival. It's like studying the cosmos: no
matter how much is viewed, no matter how much is learned, there is
always so much more! So it is not the least bit surprising to learn that,
regarding something as crucial to survival as having a steady supply of
glucose available for all the living body's needs, there are means by
which glucose can be supplied if for some reason an insufficient
amount of glucose-rich carbohydrates are not regularly consumed.

It has been well established that the three categories of food—
proteins, fats, and carbohydrates—each have their own, clearly
defined purpose with regard to the needs of the living body: protein
for the building, repair, and maintenance of tissue; fat for heat,
padding, protection of organs, and regulation of fat-soluble vitamins;

and carbohydrates for energy. However, in an emergency—in a crisis situation—if insufficient carbohydrates are consumed, for whatever reason, the body has the ability to actually convert proteins and/or fat into glucose. Amazing! There's even a word to describe the process, and of course it's another of those seven-syllable words you can throw a saddle on: gluconeogenesis. Not that it matters what it's called; let's just refer to it as GNG.

Unfortunately, this process of GNG is an extremely exhaustive and demanding one and is enormously taxing for the body. The living body will *only* resort to it if it sees itself as threatened, at which point it enters into the same state as it would if being starved. Faced with starvation, the body has no choice: it does what it has to do to survive. There's no question that the body *can* perform this complex process under dire circumstances, but why force it to do so and push it to the brink where it actually feels threatened? To do so consistently as a lifestyle can only have long-term catastrophic repercussions.

I know there are those people who declare that the body will routinely extract its glucose needs either from metabolized carbohydrates or from stored fat through the process of GNG as if it made no difference which source is used. But by any standard of reason, logic, common sense, intelligence, or the power of deduction, such a suggestion is ludicrous, to put it mildly. As if the body thinks, *Well, let's see. I obtained my glucose needs from carbohydrates yesterday. I think I'll tap them from fat today—just to switch it up a bit; keep things interesting.* That is beyond absurd. The body, according to nature's grand plan, *naturally* relies upon carbohydrates for its energy needs, not fat. The only way fat is utilized for energy is if the body is starved of carbohydrates.

I find it so fascinating that one surefire way of making a product more appealing is to slap the words "All Natural" on it. Even when the word "natural" has been so thoroughly corrupted it is barely recognizable and winds up on products no more natural than red dye #40, people are attracted to that which is natural. Well, the *natural* order of things is for the living body to obtain its energy from carbohydrates not fats; that is nature's plan! To create a situation where the body is so fearful for its well-being that it feels compelled to resort to emergency measures is not very respectful of what is normal and natural. Doing so defies nature, and in the process it forces the body to overwork and deplete its precious storehouse of metabolic enzymes unnecessarily in order to do the added work.

You may very well be thinking right now that no one would deliberately put the body through such an ordeal, but you'd be mistaken. To explain what I mean, I have to return to the subject of weight-loss diets—the unsavory side of weight-loss diets. The unfortunate truth is that there are people who know how to prey upon other people's frustration and desperation to lose weight. The sad fact is some people will try something—even something inherently dangerous—if there is even the slightest chance of losing weight.

"CARBOHYDRATES" IS *NOT* A BAD WORD!

I made the point earlier that removing any one of the three categories of food—proteins, fats, or carbohydrates—in order to lose weight, rather than consuming all three in the proper balance, and in the purest form, as part of a well-rounded, intelligent eating lifestyle, was a serious mistake that would ultimately take its toll on those who fell for such an approach to eating. One such diet rose to immense popularity in the mid- to late 1990s by an author, now deceased, whose name I prefer not to mention because, to be perfectly honest with you, I don't want his name in my book.

You see, this person realized that if the body feels threatened as a result of being starved of the carbohydrates it requires and must have on a regular basis, the result will be a loss of weight as the body burns fat for energy in order to have fuel for the brain and to survive. And he turned this dreadfully hurtful idea into the most abominable diet in all the history of abominable diets. People desperate to lose weight, who were not aware of the consequences of such an approach to eating, went on the diet to lose weight, oblivious to the catastrophic repercussions that awaited them down the road.

If I told you that the way to never ever stub your toe again is to simply cut off your foot, would you do it? Or would you wonder how I managed to get out of my straightjacket? To recommend the body be starved *intentionally* of its needed carbohydrates in order to lose weight is no better an idea, because eating in that way consistently puts one's life is in jeopardy.

People did start to lose weight, not realizing they were sacrificing long-term good health in favor of short-term weight loss. It worked by tricking the body into thinking it was sick. It actually forced the body into a sort of temporary disease state so that maintaining the weight it was carrying became secondary to survival. Have you ever seen people in the final stages of a catastrophic disease like cancer or AIDS? They are emaciated because they have no appetite for food. This is what the all-protein, no-carbohydrate diet this man came up with relied on.

When the body is in crisis—in other words, when the body is sick or its energy reserves are in short supply, as is the case when starved of carbohydrates—the intelligent living body's protective mechanism kicks in and automatically decreases the appetite in order to conserve and best utilize what energy is available. Remember, digestion gobbles up the lion's share of available energy so the less food that is eaten the more energy will be available for healing.

At the moment when the body most desperately needed the carbohydrates *naturally designed* to relieve such a situation, carbohydrates were instead forbidden in favor of huge quantities of cooked—therefore dead—animal products. The original version of this death diet, which became so popular, made it clear that if you were awake you could gorge yourself on any amount of animal products you could get into your stomach anytime, day or night. But even look at a picture of a piece of fruit and you might as well put your affairs in order and prepare to meet your maker.

I told you I would not test your patience with a bunch of physiological jibber jabber, and I'm not going to, but in order to further substantiate what I am talking about here, I need to briefly discuss

one word with you. It is a word with which you are very likely familiar: saccharide (pronounced SACK-uh-ride). Saccharide is merely
another way of saying carbohydrate. A monosaccharide contains one
molecule of carbohydrate, a disaccharide contains two molecules of
carbohydrate, and a polysaccharide contains three or more molecules
of carbohydrate.

Glucose *is* a monosaccharide. In other words, the only fuel the
human brain can burn is a monosaccharide (glucose). And until anything that is put into the body is turned into a monosaccharide, it
cannot be used by the brain. Period—end of conversation.

Here's an interesting aspect of all this that you should find
instructive. There are two foods in the human diet that are *naturally
occurring* monosaccharides—only two. The first is mother's milk.
That is certainly in alignment with the immense intelligence that
governs life. Of course Mother Nature would provide for infants a
perfectly nourishing food that requires no effort from the body to
have fuel for the brain.

The second food that is a naturally occurring monosaccharide,
which nature has provided to supply us with immediately accessible,
high-quality fuel for the brain without it having to go through any
energy-intensive processes to make it so, is . . . trumpets and drum
roll, please . . . fruit! And of course the sugar component in fruit is
fructose.

If supplied with high-quality carbohydrates in their purest form
and in a proper balance along with proteins and fats, as is part of
nature's grand plan, the living body does not have to feel threatened,
does not have to enter the starvation or disease state, does not have
to push itself to the limit, does not have to overtax its vital resources,
and does not have to throw itself into turmoil in order to survive. But
along comes our reckless friend with his "Eat all the dead animal
products you can but don't you dare eat a piece of fruit" diet, and
what is his addlebrained contribution to humankind? *Turn carbohydrates into a bad word!*

As a point of interest regarding carbohydrates and their inherent value to us humans, at what point in life do you think it would be most crucial to supply the very best, most nutritious diet possible? I would like you to consider the newborn. At no other time in life will there be such rapid and dramatic growth than there will be in the earliest stages of life. Most infants will double their birth weight by three or four months and triple their birth weight by twelve months. *Triple* their weight in only one year; now that's impressive. They had better have the ultimate food and fuel to pull that off, wouldn't you say? Who better to rely upon for the very best of the best nourishment for brand-new life than Mother Nature herself?

Fortunately, the days of new mothers being convinced to take shots in order to dry up their breast milk because formula was as good or even *better* than breast milk (and certainly more convenient) are gone and, quite frankly, good riddance. I know, I know, it sounds too bizarre to possibly be true, but that's what was going on in the 1950s and 1960s. Today it is recognized the world over that *nothing* can even come close to the perfection of breast milk. Of the three constituents of food—proteins, fats, and carbohydrates—what do you think the composition of breast milk is? Mostly protein for the building of tissue for all that rapid growth? You'd be wrong. The greatest percentage by far of breast milk is water. But of the solids, what if I told you that the protein and fat content *combined* did not equal the carbohydrate content? Breast milk is right around 1 percent protein, 4.5 percent fat, and a little over 7 percent carbohydrate. Now why do you think that is?

Now, if the fact that fruit is a monosaccharide were the one and only positive aspect of its nature, that *alone* would warrant it being given the highest priority in our diet. However, there's more—lots more. Fruit is not only naturally high in fiber but also contains crucial vitamins, minerals, enzymes, amino acids, fatty acids, phytonutrients, and antioxidants. In fact, every substance or compound known to support and promote life is resplendent in fruit.

Plus fruit is completely devoid of saturated fat and cholesterol, substances researchers the world over recommend we eat in moderation.

Cooked animal products are devoid of fiber and high in fat and cholesterol, are an *extremely* poor source of energy that in turn requires huge amounts of energy to be digested, and their nutrient content is severely compromised due to the high heat required to cook them. Overconsumption of cooked protein and fat is associated with every disease known to afflict the human population. But wait, there's more!

FRUIT: THE PERFECT ENERGY SOURCE AND ENERGY SAVER

I mentioned earlier that the digestion of food requires more energy than all other uses of energy combined. Well, guess what one food in the human diet requires virtually *no* digestion in the stomach? Right you are—fruit! Fruit passes relatively quickly through the stomach and is digested in the intestines where it releases all of its goodness. So, not only is fruit transformed into utilizable energy faster and more efficiently than any other food, it requires the least amount of energy *from* the body for it to be metabolized.

These facts clearly reveal fruit to be a most healthful and beneficial food in the human diet, *when properly eaten*. When I emphasize properly eaten, or correctly eaten, I am referring to fruit's unique nature of not requiring digestion in the stomach. There is a right way and a wrong way to eat fruit to benefit from its goodness, and it's led to so much misinformation about its consumption. I will discuss shortly the optimum way to eat fruit so you can reap its many rewards and avoid any potential pitfalls.

Considering that fruit fulfills the requirements for nutrients and energy more fully and perfectly than any other food, could it not reasonably be expected to comprise a significant part of our diet? Instead it has traditionally been viewed as a once in a while treat and is all too frequently used merely for ornamental purposes.

Before we go on to discuss how to eat fruit for optimal health, let me finish the story I started earlier about the famous dead-food diet.

Mercifully, this antilife, body-abusing, brain-torturing diet ran its course. As more and more people noticed that their breath smelled like a broken sewer line, and as lawsuits and hundreds of complaints were lodged against it for the health problems it caused, and while doctors, dieticians, and nutritionists (the sane ones anyway) railed against it relentlessly, people finally got the picture.

Of course the death of the diet's author also put a serious crimp in the credibility of his diet. Even though a lame attempt was made to attribute his death to the complications resulting from a bump on the head received in a fall on an icy sidewalk, someone obtained a copy of his autopsy report and released it to the public and that, as they say, was that. Not only was he clinically obese at the time of his death, but he also had high blood pressure, an enlarged heart, clogged arteries, and congestive heart failure. In other words, this man's heart and cardiovascular system were in deplorable condition, and it was his antilife diet that put it in that state.

THE BEST WAY TO EAT FRUIT

Let's move on to something far more positive and enjoyable shall we: fruit eatin'. The difference between fruit being eaten to dramatically improve your health and well-being while assisting your efforts to lose weight and it being a destructive force that causes problems and hinders your weight-loss efforts is one simple factor: eating fruit correctly.

Whatever could I mean by "eating fruit correctly"? Wouldn't picking up a piece of fruit, biting into it, chewing it, and swallowing it be eating fruit correctly? Yes, it would, in so far as the mechanical phase of getting the fruit into your body is concerned. However, I am referring to the *physiological* aspect of fruit eating. Just a moment ago, while discussing all of the positive features of fruit, I pointed out the fact that fruit is the one food in the human diet that does not require digestion in the stomach; fruit passes through the stomach and is digested in the intestines. Therefore: *Eating fruit correctly*

means eating it alone, fresh, and on an empty stomach, not with or fol-
lowing any other food.

Learning this simple, yet immensely profound, dietary reality has had a greater positive impact on my health and well-being than any other dietary principle I have ever learned in my decades of study. And judging from the feedback received from those who have followed *Fit For Life* over the years, the same is true for millions of others. I only hope you are able to see the virtue of what I am imparting here so you too can reap the numerous rewards in store for you by eating fruit correctly.

To honor fruit's unique nature in our diet, it is imperative it not be impeded in any way from passing straight through the stomach into the intestines—where all its benefits can be realized. Forcing fruit to stay in the stomach where it doesn't belong and is not intended to be causes a host of problems for the body that are both painful and energy depleting.

Fruit's journey through the stomach *will* be thwarted if, one, there is other food already in the stomach, or, two, if the fruit is eaten along with other foods that require digestion in the stomach. When this happens and fruit is forced to stay in the stomach where it encounters digestive juices, it immediately ferments and spoils. That in turn causes whatever starches are in the stomach to ferment and whatever proteins are there to putrefy. It's a mess, and all the positives associated with eating fruit correctly are lost and are instead turned into negatives.

Fruit, like all living foods, already contains all the necessary enzymes it needs for its digestion. No digestive enzymes have to be produced by the body (as is the case with cooked foods) *provided* the fruit enzymes are not destroyed by heat. If the fruit is canned, or otherwise cooked or pasteurized, that fruit is dead and will be forced to stay in the stomach where digestive enzymes will have to be made available. You know what that means: the metabolic enzyme storehouse is forced to give up some of its precious payload.

BALANCE IS THE KEY

Another important aspect of correctly eating fruit is associated with the acid-alkaline balance in the body referred to as the pH balance. It is likely you are at least familiar enough with this feature of the living body to know that being too acidic is not in the best interest of your health and well-being. Acidic diets, which most diets are, cause the body to use up calcium and other minerals in order to help neutralize acid. Also, the body retains water to try to dilute acid and that leads to weight gain.

The pH balance of the body is measured on a scale of 0 to 14, with 0 representing pure acid, 14 representing pure alkaline, and 7 as neutral. The healthy bloodstream is approximately 7.35 to 7.45 on the pH scale. In other words, your blood is slightly alkaline, and your health depends upon it remaining so. As you can see, the desirable range is exceedingly small. So small, in fact, that if your blood were to reach even the neutral point of 7, you would become extremely sick, and it could even be fatal for you.

Here's an interesting fact about fruit that most people don't know: *all* fruit is alkaline and therefore helps neutralize acid in the body. I know what you're thinking: *Hey, what about oranges, grapefruits, pineapples, and lemons. They're not alkaline, they're acid fruits, right?* Sort of. Their classification as acid fruits is only their *botanical* classification. Once inside the body, however, all fruit is alkaline, *unless* it has been subjected to heat, either by cooking or pasteurization, or by coming into contact with food in the stomach. Then it is acid and it *stays* acid, and contributes greatly to the problems associated with a predominantly acid-producing diet.

Once heated by any means or forced to stay in the stomach with other foods, fruit and fruit juice go from being one of the most important and effective tools you have in maintaining your weight and well-being to yet one more factor in the decline of your overall health. What a tragedy. Here is a food, a delicious and healthy food at that, being largely misunderstood, ignored, and unappreciated simply because of too much misinformation and a lack of good information. That needn't be the case for you any longer.

The Best Way to Drink Fruit Juice

Fruit juices can be a marvelous addition to your diet, as they assist the body in cleansing while supplying high-quality nutrition as well as the most supreme energy source. But once again, juices, just like the whole fruit, must be consumed correctly. I truly wish it were otherwise, but the vast majority of juices people drink are not only worthless but also harmful. Do you know why? They're pasteurized. Heat kills. In this case, as stated earlier, at 118°F all the enzymes are destroyed and what is being consumed is a pleasant *tasting* juice that is pure acid in the body.

All those bottles and cartons of juice with pretty pictures on them declaring them to be fresh and natural are neither fresh nor natural. Marketers will use terms like "Made With Real Juice," and that may be true; they *started* with something real, but wound up with something real bad for you. Fresh orange juice may be one of the most perfect liquids you can drink, but when pasteurized it is so acidic in the body it can literally burn a hole in your stomach (otherwise known as an ulcer) or severely aggravate an existing ulcer. Seriously, you would be so much better off drinking water or nothing at all rather than drinking fruit juice that has been pasteurized, and that includes juices made from concentrate, all of which are pasteurized.

Here's another tip about drinking juice. People have a tendency to gulp juices down. Quite frankly, that's not a real good idea. It's best to drink juice slowly—one mouthful at a time—giving it a chance mix with saliva. Drinking juice this way won't overwhelm your stomach with too much too soon. All of the potential negatives associated with fruit and fruit juices can be avoided, and all the potential benefits they have to offer can be fully realized, simply by consuming them in the manner in which nature intended: alone and fresh—not processed, refined, heated, or altered from their natural state.

THE GOOD, THE BAD, AND THE UGLY ABOUT FRUCTOSE

Life is full of ironies. Some are so peculiar as to make reasonable thinking people scratch their heads in bewilderment. Over the last forty-plus years during which I have been studying the principles of good health, there is one irony that is so bizarre it has made me scratch my head almost to the point of bleeding. I know that name-calling is the last recourse of an exhausted mind, but some of the unbridled ignorance associated with how bad fruit and fruit juices are because of their sugar component (fructose) *really* push me to the limit of civility. How in the name of all that is life giving could the one food on the planet that has the greatest potential for good over any other in the human diet, have developed such a totally unjustified and inaccurate reputation? It brings to mind the now-famous quote by none other than Mark Twain: "A truth is not hard to kill but a lie told well is immortal."

I know there are some people who will never, *ever* accept what I am going to say here about fructose because they have a permanent, unalterable blind spot or have too much of a vested interest in the stance they have championed over the years. Their egos simply won't allow them to acknowledge that they had it wrong. Fine. I'm no longer trying to convince those folks. My goal is to prevent you, dear reader, from falling into the trap of accepting as accurate, erroneous information from the people who know a whole lot about what ain't so.

Have you ever heard of the Piccadilly Circus? Do you think there are any elephants or clowns there? Well there aren't. The Piccadilly Circus is a public circle in London's West End where five of the city's busiest streets converge, and there's plenty of shopping but no circus animals or clowns. In this instance, circus doesn't mean circus in the traditional sense. It's just a word and can obviously have two meanings.

"Fructose" is just a word. It's what we *attach* to the word that gives it meaning. And what has been attached to the word "fructose" is pure sophistry—an argument that *seems* plausible but is actually dishonest and misleading. It is a classic example of using a half-truth to convince someone into believing something that would be rejected straight away were the entire truth known. I am not implying that the people who speak negatively about fructose are doing so maliciously. I don't think they are. I think they simply don't understand the difference inside the living body of a substance that is in its natural state and one that has been deranged or otherwise altered from its natural state. How many times have you heard something to the effect of "it's the simplest things in life that we often miss"? That is what I think we are dealing with here.

The argument against fructose is rooted in that same tired old standard of "sugar is sugar." It can be the sugar in a candy bar or the sugar in a peach; it just doesn't make any difference in the body, where chemically they're the same. This argument is *so* weak, so fallacious, I'm almost embarrassed to have to take it any more seriously than if I was reading it in *MAD* magazine. It reminds me of when I was in high school and some practical joker would tell me something totally ludicrous with a completely deadpan, straight face just to see if I would fall for it so everyone could have a good laugh at my expense.

That same "sugar is sugar" argument was used to push calorie counting: a calorie is a calorie in the body because they're both the same measure of heat. But that was finally acknowledged to be erroneous thinking. Logically, it just didn't hold up to scrutiny. The factor that had to be taken into consideration was what was the quality of the package that transported the calorie into the body? After all, calories brought into the body from a bag of potato chips are not going to be as healthy overall as those transported into the body by a fresh vegetable salad.

It's the same with the example I gave earlier about water. Chemically, water is H_2O, yes, but the point was made that a glass of mountain spring water consumed on a regular basis will be a great boon to the body, whereas ocean water consumed on a regular basis will result in death. It doesn't matter if both are chemically H_2O in the body.

I made a similar point when I talked about the grain of wheat taken from ancient tombs that sprouted when put into soil versus the freshly harvested grain of wheat that was heated (in other words, killed) and would *not* sprout. They were both grains of wheat, but there was one big difference, wasn't there? The one that sprouted had the benefit of still containing the life force within it, whereas the one that did not sprout was lacking that all-important intangible: life!

One of those areas of complete agreement within the health community is that refined sugar is a killer. I don't feel the need to go into details here, except to say that refined sugar is a major contributor to so many health problems it would take a separate book to list them all: heart and other cardiovascular diseases, cancer, liver disease, diabetes, arthritis, osteoporosis, obesity—the list is interminable. It is a sad state of affairs, but refined sugar, in a variety of forms, is being sneaked into your food in such dizzying amounts that the average person now consumes 180 pounds per year! Ouch!

Sometime in the 1970s the food and beverage manufacturers discovered a sweetener usually derived from corn called high-fructose corn syrup (HFCS). What they liked most about it is that it is far less expensive to make than regular old table sugar (sucrose) and about 20 percent sweeter. This was great, financially speaking, but it has taken a devastating toll on the health of those who consume it regularly. And you know what usually transpires when financial gain is measured against the risk to the consumer's health, don't you? There was no contest. When it came time to decide whether or not to go forward with HFCS, it was "Katie bar the door, we're going full-speed ahead." This is not a time for tiptoeing around the issue or politically correct niceties; HFCS is an abomination. Anyone who would attempt to convince you otherwise is either woefully ill informed, or lying. Both adults and children alike are dealing with unprecedented obesity and overweight challenges and HFCS is in no small part to blame. I readily acknowledge that there are other factors contributing to this sorrowful reality but since the advent of HFCS, these weight-related statistics have skyrocketed.

How Drug Makers Use Half-Truths to Sell You Drugs

The number of drugs being prescribed these days is a national disgrace. I know there are instances when drugs have their place—emergency situations require emergency measures. I know that. But the fact that there is the equivalent of *twelve* prescriptions for drugs written for every man, woman, and child in the United States reveals that there is a bit too much drug pushing going on. And this does not even include millions of over-the-counter drugs! Some very clever marketing strategies must be employed to convince the beleaguered consumer to take more and more drugs, and the strategy of choice is the half-truth.

Have you ever heard of statins? They have been referred to as "the latest miracle drug" or "the new aspirin." What they are is the pharmaceutical industry's goldmine. Tens of billions of dollars worth are sold a year. Statins are dangerous drugs that in addition to causing standard, run-of-the-mill side effects like headache, nausea, constipation, and weakness, also cause severe pain and weakness of the muscles, liver damage, kidney failure, digestive difficulties, memory loss, and heart and other cardiovascular problems. They are prescribed for the lowering of cholesterol. Most people are aware of the fact that an overabundance of cholesterol in the body can lead to some major health problems. That's the half of the truth that the pharmaceutical industry focuses on.

Some people are still confused about where cholesterol comes from, which is surprising since it comes from only *one place* in the universe and absolutely nowhere else. Cholesterol is produced in the livers of animals.

Trying to lose weight while consuming HFCS is like trying to sober up while drinking whiskey. When HFCS enters the body, it makes a beeline for the liver where it is immediately turned to fat. Unlike other carbohydrates that trigger the pancreas to secrete insulin, which signals appetite suppression to the brain, HFCS *hinders* the natural production of insulin. So not only does it quickly turn to fat but it also stops you from feeling full.

In fact, we human beings produce somewhere between 1,000 and 2,000 mg of cholesterol every day. That is because cholesterol is an *absolute necessity of life.* That's the half the pharmaceutical industry conveniently leaves out. Practically every function of the body, from blinking the eyes to swallowing, from walking to internal functions, requires cholesterol. However, it's not the cholesterol the body produces for its own use and well-being that presents any problem; it's the cholesterol from other animals we eat that is the culprit.

Statins work by inhibiting the liver's ability to produce cholesterol. So the cholesterol that is beneficial and uniquely designed for the human body, and which is an indispensable factor in health and well-being is *suppressed,* and the cholesterol that is harmful and dangerous that we obtain from the overconsumption of animal products is allowed to circulate in the bloodstream. That's just wrong!

Plus, there is another vital substance produced in the liver that is crucial for good heart health—coenzyme Q10 (CoQ10), also called "ubiquinol." Statins also inhibit the production of this crucial enzyme. The insufferable irony here is that people have been convinced to purchase a very expensive drug that thwarts the production of vital, naturally occurring substances while putting their health—their very life—at risk. And all the while the best way to reduce the *foreign, damaging* cholesterol is simply to eat fewer animal products.

The stance of those who push statins on people is totally one-pointed: cholesterol bad. That's half true: the cholesterol from the overeating of animal products is indeed bad, but the cholesterol manufactured by the living body for its own well-being is not only good, it's essential.

Today, so many packaged and processed foods contain the stuff it's almost easier to list which ones do not. It's in sodas (by far one of the worst offenders) and other sweetened beverages like iced tea and fake fruit juices, dressings, breakfast cereals, candy, ketchup and other tomato-based sauces like spaghetti, barbeque, and pizza sauces, many packaged meals like macaroni and cheese, bread and other baked goods, ice cream, yogurt, cookies and crackers, pretzels, numerous items at fast food outlets, soups, and a host of other foods too numerous to list. Even some supposedly "natural" items like "healthy" granola bars contain HFCS as do jams, jellies, and syrups; many brands of the most popular maple syrup, even ones declared to be "real" maple syrup, are nothing more than HFCS with added maple syrup "flavor." Start reading ingredient labels—you will be shocked when you see how frequently HFCS shows up.

Unfortunately, as the damage caused by HFCS began to be more apparent, some members of the health community started in with the old refrain: "Fructose in *any* form is bad—fructose is fructose." Good grief, not again! HFCS or a fresh piece of fruit? It makes no difference to the Chicken Littles. Never mind that one can wreak havoc in the body while the other is a naturally occurring monosaccharide that can be efficiently used in the body. All "they" know is that the sky is falling: fructose is fructose!

It's the same old half-truth strategy being employed yet again. And half-truths like these can have a catastrophic effect on your health. The pharmaceutical industry in particular utilizes this half-truth, propaganda-like tactic more than any other industry I can think of. (See "How Drug Makers Use Half-Truths to Sell You Drugs" on page 108.)

The stance of those who disparage fructose is also one-pointed: fructose bad. That's only half true. The fructose in HFCS—which is in no way natural, has been processed and refined, deranged by heat, had its molecular structure altered, had all of its enzymes and other nutritional elements destroyed, been subjected to chemicals, and no longer exists in the context of a whole food—is indeed bad. Terrible, in fact.

The fructose in a fresh piece of fruit, eaten *correctly*, is living, has its enzyme component intact, has not been heated, has not been treated with chemicals, has not been processed or in any other way altered from its natural condition, and is easily and efficiently utilized by the living body, and it is supremely good for you.

There is one more subtle, exceedingly important aspect of this discussion, perhaps *too* subtle to be grasped by those who are over-thinking this issue. The fructose in a living piece of fresh fruit, designed by nature itself, exists within a harmonious framework with all the other constituents of the food in which it is grown. There are two points associated with this fact that simply cannot be overemphasized but are unfortunately being overlooked:

1. The fructose has not been heated or altered from its molecular structure in *any* way. It has not been deranged. *IT HAS NOT BEEN REFINED!* And as was pointed out in the previous chapter the refining process is the death knell for any food.

2. Perhaps most important of all, the fructose has not been extracted and fragmented—*it has not been isolated*—but rather is utilized in concert with all of the other elements of the food.

Regarding this second point, not all of the elements that exist in food are even known. Nor are all the processes involved in metabolizing it known. There are things going on within the living body as it interacts with whole living food that are unknown to us in the same way it is unknown to us how the living body turns an apple into blood.

Remember the two seeds of wheat I talked about earlier? One was heated and the other was not. Placed side by side, you could not tell the difference between the two. Yet when they are placed into the soil, *only* the seed that has not been heated will germinate and become a plant. Did the soil somehow "know" which one would sprout and which one wouldn't? Or was there something inherently "right" about the unheated seed that allowed it to interact with the soil and grow?

When fructose is in its pristine, unadulterated form, such as in a piece of fresh fruit, and it is correctly consumed, it is utilized by the body as a perfect source of energy or is stored as glycogen for later use. When fructose in its deranged form, such as in HFCS and is consumed, the body views it as a poison and takes whatever steps necessary to see that it is eliminated before it can cause harm. Just as the unheated wheat seed is able to interact with the soil and turn into a plant, the unadulterated fructose is able to be utilized by the body and turned into usable energy with no negative effects. To equate the fructose (or what's left of it) that is in HFCS to the fructose in a whole, fresh, living piece of fruit would be the same as equating drowning to swimming because both take place in water.

The mere inference that the exquisitely intelligent living body, capable of highly sophisticated activities that baffle the greatest minds of science, could somehow be so stupid as to be unable to distinguish a sugar that is poisonous from one that is beneficial is so patently absurd that it does not even warrant serious attention. If you were trekking through the desert with no water and you came upon two waterholes, one sparkling, clear, and fresh, the other rancid, filthy, and stinking, do you think you might be able to tell which one you would want to drink from and which one you would not?

This is so elemental that I can't believe I have to defend such feeble, unfounded arguments against fruit and its sugar component. I feel like I'm stuck in one of those old episodes of *The Twilight Zone* where I have to prove that the moon isn't made of green cheese or I'll be banished. Commercially processed sweeteners like HFCS and other artificial sweeteners like aspartame, neotame, and sucralose are poisons in the body. They're deadly. No right-thinking person can equate something that is completely artificial to something that is completely real as is the sugar in whole fruit. C'mon! One is artificial, the other is real! If you went into a bank to cash a check and were given Monopoly money, what would you think about that? Would you simply accept it, thank the teller, and leave? Or would you look around with a skeptical smile and ask if you were on *Candid Camera*?

Fructose in fresh fruit, *eaten correctly,* is utilized by the body and is of inestimable value as a source of fuel energy. I have a little proposition for those whose clarion call is, "My mind is made up, don't confuse me with the facts." How about from now on, anything you wish to purchase, no matter what it is, must be done so with diamonds. But any funds due you, in any amount from any source, will be paid to you with chunks of coal. This should present no problem for you since both are made of carbon. And after all, carbon is carbon!

EATING FRUIT AND YOUR BODY'S THREE NATURAL CYCLES

I wish to share with you the best way to eat fruit correctly and be certain you obtain its maximum benefit, as well as the reasoning behind doing so. When I first introduced the process of metabolism in the opening of the book, I pointed out that we will each consume approximately seventy tons of food in our lifetime, and I described the dynamic of taking in food, extracting and assimilating what the body needs from that food, and removing from the body the waste that is generated. It's a three-step process of eating, extracting what is needed, and eliminating the waste. Intricately intertwined with these three metabolic processes is a phenomenon I first introduced in the original *Fit For Life*, and, because of its relevance, spoke of in three subsequent books as well.

I am referring to our body's natural body cycles, or what are referred to as circadian rhythms. Each of the three processes of metabolism just so happen to correspond to three regularly recurring eight-hour cycles of physiological activities in the human body that occur every twenty-four hours. Our body cycles represent the elegance, synergy, and interconnectedness of the intelligence that governs our existence.

The eight-hour body cycle that coincides with eating is called the *appropriation cycle*. It is operational from approximately 12 noon until 8:00 pm and represents the time during which it is most advantageous to take in food. The eight-hour body cycle that coincides with the extraction of nutrients and energy sources is called the *assimilation cycle*. It is operational from approximately 8:00 pm until 4:00

am, and it is when the body is extracting and absorbing what it needs. The eight-hour body cycle that coincides with the elimination of waste is called the *elimination cycle*. It is operational from approximately 4:00 am until 12 noon, and it is when the eliminative processes of the body are at their most heightened.

It's not that complicated, is it? We eat (appropriation), we take from the food what is needed (assimilation), and we remove the waste (elimination). In terms of being successful in losing weight *and* in optimizing health, we want to pay special attention to the elimination cycle. The reason is that anything in the body that is not contributing to overall well-being and is instead impeding the body's efforts to function optimally needs to be removed. This is the key to your success in any effort to lose weight. Therefore, it only makes good sense that whatever is in your power to do in order to streamline and optimize the activities of your elimination cycle should be undertaken. Conversely, anything you are doing that burdens or interferes with the elimination cycle should be discontinued or at the very least minimized.

Usually, when someone thinks of elimination from the body the first thing that comes to mind are bowel movements. And without a doubt that is one of the four primary means of elimination, along with the bladder, the millions of pores of the skin, and every exhaled breath. However, the elimination cycle is so very much more than bringing wastes to the four channels of elimination. It is responsible for first collecting the waste that is produced individually by every one of the 100 trillion cells of the body spoken of earlier.

You should be clear that when I refer to the time during which the elimination cycle is operational—4:00 am to 12 noon—that is not to imply that at exactly 4:00 am the elimination cycle starts up and at exactly 12 noon it closes down. Eliminating wastes from the body is so enormously crucial to life that, to some degree, it is going on at all times (as are the other two cycles). However, elimination is most heightened during the hours of 4:00 am until 12 noon.

We already know that there isn't an activity of the body that does not require some energy. Since there is only a certain amount of energy to go around, obviously the more activities there are drawing on that energy, the less there will be for the others.

As discussed earlier in the book, the one activity of the body that gobbles up more energy than any other is digestion. So clearly, when there is no digestion going on in the stomach, the other activities of the body, including, of course, the body cycles, have access to what energy is available. And since food in the stomach is a priority for the body, the moment food enters the stomach, whatever energy is needed is diverted there regardless of other activities that may have to be temporarily shortchanged.

To illustrate what I'm talking about, let's say you wake up at 8:00 am and have breakfast, which is customary in most places in the world. Well, 8:00 am is exactly in the middle and at the height of the elimination cycle. Having breakfast, which fires up the digestive process, slams the brakes on the elimination cycle. That is not something you want to do every day of your life if losing weight is a concern for you. There are people, some of whom are reading this right now, who have eaten breakfast every day of their life, which means that not once, not *ever*, has their elimination cycle been allowed to operate unfettered from beginning to end.

I can just hear some people saying right now, "Whoa, brother. If you're suggesting what I *think* you're suggesting, I'm giving this book to my dog to gnaw on. Don't even think of telling me I have to give up eating breakfast." I'm not—not exactly anyway. Look, I am all too familiar, as I'm sure you are, with the relentlessly repeated admonitions that "breakfast is the most important meal of the day" and "you have to eat a good, hearty breakfast for energy." That is advice that comes from marketers representing big business and from the ill-informed, not from anyone who has even an inkling of an idea that there is any such thing as an elimination cycle.

Before I reveal what I'm going to propose to you, I really have to explain why the statement that a hearty breakfast is necessary for energy is an ill-informed thing to say. After a typical breakfast you don't feel energized, you feel tired; and the more food eaten the more tired you are. You know what I'm saying is true from your own experience. Why? Because turning food into energy isn't something that happens quickly—it takes *hours*. And, as we know, it actually *requires* energy to perform the process of turning glucose *into* energy. The actual energy you will be operating on during the day was built the night before while you were asleep.

When you awaken in the morning, your body has been busy through the night producing the energy you will need during the day. Sitting down to a "hearty breakfast" is going to gobble up a good portion of that energy. Have you ever heard the term "midmorning slump"? Why do you think drinking caffeinated beverages is a national pastime in this country? The digestion of food requires a lot of energy and makes you tired!

I know it is a perfectly reasonable thing to think that by eating breakfast, the energy from that meal will provide energy later in the day. But what will you be doing about four hours or so after you finished breakfast? Having lunch! Now remember, breakfast had to be in your stomach for approximately three hours before it could even leave the stomach and *start* the process of being transformed into energy. But a new meal, lunch, hits the stomach for *its* three-hour stay. And what will you be doing four or five hours after lunch? Here it comes—having dinner! Another three-hour, energy-usurping meal.

Let me ask you a question. As the day proceeds, do you have more energy? Or do you grow tired and just want to relax? The idea of eating a hearty breakfast for energy throughout the day seems reasonable to those who are unaware of what you have just read here, but in actual fact you need to have a good night's sleep to have energy for your next day's activities. And waking up in the morning and spending a good chunk of it on breakfast is *not* the best way to start the day.

I said the "typical" breakfast doesn't energize you, but there is one type of breakfast that does. Can you guess what it is? What is the one food that requires *no* digestive energy in the stomach? What is the one food that is a naturally occurring monosaccharide so it is transformed into usable energy quicker and more efficiently than any other? It's not bacon and eggs, my friend; you know I am referring to the perfect food—fruit.

Eat Fruit for Breakfast!

Here is my recommendation to you for when you wake in the morning and want to optimize, not squander, the energy built during the night. From the time you awaken until 12 noon eat only fruit. You can have as much as you want, as frequently as you want throughout the morning—so long as it is fresh. Same thing if you want orange juice; it must be fresh, not pasteurized. By having only fruit you will not be using up the energy needed for the elimination cycle, which also runs until 12 noon. You can have whole pieces of fruit, dried fruit, fruit salad, fruit juice, or fruit smoothies.

I have been making this recommendation to people for forty years. I have been following the advice myself during that time. No other dietary practice I've learned has had a greater or more profound impact on my health and well-being than having fruit until noon. Some people will find this easier to do than others, but I hope it makes enough sense to you that you at least *try* it for a while to see if what I am saying is true.

I could easily give you hundreds of examples of people over the years who told me, sometimes tearfully, that they loved fruit and really wanted to eat it, but they didn't for the longest time because of the pain and discomfort they experienced. But after learning that fruit eaten with other foods or as dessert after a big meal was the cause of their difficulties, they started eating it correctly—fresh, alone, and on an empty stomach—and as though by magic they were able to enjoy fruit again with no problems.

One woman told me that she had not had a glass of orange juice for over ten years because of the excruciating pain it caused her. After learning about why this happened—that it was because it was pasteurized and frequently consumed with or after other foods—she started drinking it unpasteurized and on an empty stomach, and it never again gave her any problem.

I know that if this is a new concept for you the idea of having only fruit until noon can initially be a daunting, even shocking, prospect. Please understand that this is not some intractable edict that must be followed or all is lost. It's not as though your weight-loss efforts, including taking Slender GR™, will not work for you unless you eat fruit until noon, because that's not the case. I am merely striving to give you some well-proven tools you can use in your life that stand all on their own and will help you achieve your weight and health goals if you will just try them.

Perhaps you want to have fruit until noon on some days and not on others. Or maybe instead of going until noon every day, on some days you only want to go to 10:00 or 11:00, or as close to noon as is comfortable for you. Fine! Make it work for you; fit it into your lifestyle so it is convenient, not stressful. As I've said, it's not a contest. It's just about you trying to make life more satisfying and fulfilling. And another advantage to eating fruit until noon to whatever degree you do, is that it ups the amount of living food in your diet.

Obviously you are interested in doing something for yourself or you would not be reading this right now. Try this: run a test on yourself for ten days. Without making any other dietary changes whatsoever—none—have only fruit until noon for the next ten days, and then on day eleven go back to whatever type breakfast you were accustomed to having. See how you feel. See what your energy level is like during those days when you have fruit and on the days you don't. Just one caveat: if you do take me up on this ten-day challenge, be sure that day eleven falls on a day when you'll be able to lie around and not do much.

FRUIT-EATING TIPS FOR SPECIAL SITUATIONS

There are some people who do not work traditional 9-to-5 hours, and they wonder about the body cycles and how eating fruit in the

Fruit-Eating Guidelines for Diabetics

If you are diabetic or diabetes prone, you will understandably want to know how eating fruit will affect that condition. Of all the maladies that can occur in human beings, diabetes is without a doubt the *most* troublesome and challenging due to the numerous unknown variables that can come into play with this condition for each individual. What I can tell you is this: some people with diabetes have done very well eating fruit (correctly, of course), and others have not. I wish I knew the answer to why that is but I don't and that's just me being honest with you.

All you can do is follow the recommendations while keeping a close eye on your condition and see which category you are in. I wish I had something more to offer, but diabetes has been a great enigma for the scientific community and me for decades. As much as I would like to, it is nearly impossible to give a recommendation as to how much fruit you should eat without very close monitoring, which I am obviously not able to do. That will have to fall on the shoulders of your healthcare provider. I have noticed that those with type-2 diabetes have a much easier time of it when it comes to eating fruit—*correctly*, of course. But even those with type 1 have had some success.

morning will work for them. The human body is amazingly adaptable and will acclimate itself to your schedule if you are consistent. Consistency is the key. The important thing is to eat fruit and juice for several hours upon awakening, whenever that is. Also, try to allow about three hours to elapse after eating before you go to sleep (the only exception would be for eating fruit). It has been the experience of those who work the "swing shift" or "graveyard shift" that the more living food dominates the diet overall, the better they feel.

Remember when I was talking about the fact that a normal and natural part of living is the generation of toxins in the body, and that it is the lymph system's job to remove them before they cause harm? When one alters the diet in a way that frees up energy—such as by eating fruit properly and properly combining proteins and starches—

the intelligent body diverts that newfound energy to the cleansing of toxins and that can sometimes be uncomfortable. It doesn't always happen and it doesn't happen to everyone. But during the first few days, if you should feel "out of sorts" or get a headache or other body aches, or a runny nose, please don't be alarmed. Just continue what you are doing and know that the body will acclimate itself to the influx of newfound energy and things will normalize. I know those things can be uncomfortable, but on the positive side, it shows how responsive your body is to ridding itself of toxins—and that is a good thing!

Over the years, I have had the opportunity to meet and communicate with more people than I can count. It has given me an extremely large reservoir of experiences with people and with their similarities and differences as regards the effect of diet on their physiology. I have often said, and it is my belief, that no one approach to diet is right for every person. I *can* say with confidence, and I believe it to be so, that every living being on earth would benefit from an increase in living food. However, as to what particular foods and in what quantities and at what time they are eaten, experience has shown me that making universal, blanket statements is not realistic. There will always be someone who will not "fit the mold."

Teeccino Instead of Coffee

For those of you who recognize that coffee is not something that is as good for you as you would like for it to be, but like having it nonetheless, I have some great news for you. Teeccino (pronounced tih-CHEE-no) is a caffeine-free, organic, herbal coffee blend of herbs, nuts, fruits, chicory root, and grains that looks, tastes, and brews exactly like coffee without any of the negative side effects. Plus, it is not acidic in the body. Coffee aficionados rave about Teeccino's full-bodied, dark-roasted flavor and many cannot tell the difference between the two. I'm not a coffee drinker myself, but people who are have told me that this coffee alternative really delivers.

There was a time when I was certain that anyone and everyone would do well on the fruit until noon method of eating. I was mistaken. Now, to be sure, the vast, *vast* majority of people do fare extremely well eating fruit until noon—definitely over 90 percent. But there are people who, for whatever reason, do not flourish as do most people. It has something to do with their body's particular insulin response to sugar and their blood sugar levels. I don't pretend to have all the answers or to understand every nuance of the body dynamic, all I can do is try to understand as much as I can and rely on my decades-long body of experiences.

For the small segment of the population who simply cannot eat only fruit until noon and must have other food—vegetables, protein, whatever—I do wish to make one recommendation. Upon awakening in the morning have some fresh fruit or fresh fruit juice first, before you have anything else. If you can only have fruit for the first hour, so be it. If you can go a little longer, better yet. Go for as long as is comfortable and then have whatever you desire. The reason I ask this of you is so that the very first thing that enters your living body each day is something living. Recognize that you are a living being on a living planet, and let it be an acknowledgement of life by showing the appreciation you have for the living body that is looking out for your best interests every second of every day and night.

One other thing: I know there will be those of you who will say something to the effect of, "Hey, what about my morning cup of coffee?" I'm not going to lie to you. Coffee is not the best thing to have in the morning. It's a very acidic drink, and if it's caffeinated, it's even more troublesome. However, if you're going to have that one cup, again, have it an hour or so *after* you have had something living—fruit! Let the first thing you put into your body each day be something living.

• • •

It's no accident that this is the longest chapter in the book, by far. That is because I know right down to my bone marrow that if you will come to see the virtues of eating fruit correctly, and give it the importance in your life it most assuredly deserves, you will surely be rewarded. More than any other dietary principle I've ever learned, this is the one that has the potential to transform your life in ways you cannot even imagine. I know there are detractors who will disagree with my stance on fruit and that's okay: it comes with the territory when trying to impart information not familiar to the majority.

I wonder if you recognize the name Giordano Bruno? He was a spectacularly brilliant philosopher, mathematician, and astronomer. Books have been written about him, statues erected, and monuments built in his honor. Years before Galileo ever looked through a telescope, Giordano Bruno was describing the universe with astounding accuracy. The Catholic Church found his knowledge of the cosmos objectionable and so imprisoned him for seven years before having him taken out and burned to death. Among the numerous quotes attributed to this colossal luminary is the following:

> It is proof of a base and low mind for one to wish to think with the masses or majority, merely because the majority is the majority. Truth does not change because it is, or is not, believed by a majority of the people.

I really don't mind having detractors nipping at my heels, and I'll tell you why. I have something they do not have: evidence—the kind of evidence that is not easy to come by but is supremely convincing. Since 1986 I have received somewhere between 600,000 and 750,000 letters from people who have read my books, which have sold over 13 million copies. While working with a successful, professional marketing firm I was once told that because books are passed around and shared with family, friends, neighbors, and coworkers, you can multiply by two and a half the number of books sold, and that will reflect how many people likely read the book. Two and a half times 13 million is over 32 million.

I was further told that only a small percentage of people actually take the time to sit down and write an author with their feelings about what they've read. According to marketing statistics, the number of written comments received represents just a tad under 5 percent of those who feel similarly. So if 100 people write a letter, that means about 2,000 people had similar sentiments. Based on the letters I've received, that would mean about 12 to 15 million people have had experiences similar to those who wrote. That's a lot of folks. Let's say that those statistics are off by 75 percent. That would still mean somewhere between 3 and 4 million people have shared similar experiences.

Guess what one subject was, far and away, mentioned more than any other? It has been about their experience with eating fruit correctly. The comments poured in and they have not stopped. It's been over a quarter of a century since the release of the original *Fit For Life* and a week does not pass that I don't receive mail from someone saying how they have been following the principles laid out in the book for ten, fifteen, even twenty years. And even though they will sometimes go through periods of poor dietary choices, they make a point of saying that the one thing they adhere to without fail is having fruit until noon because of the transformation it brought about and the difference it made in their lives.

I know it will sound like I am exaggerating but I have personally read tens of thousands of letters from people blessing the day they learned about how to eat fruit correctly. Even people who were skeptics at first and grudgingly tried having only fruit until noon just to appease a loved one or friend wound up swearing by it. Most are genuinely astonished at how much more energy they have. So many people can't be wrong.

It would be one thing if we were talking about only a handful of people (or only a few hundred or even a few thousand people) who raved about the positive changes brought about by eating fruit correctly, but we are talking about a truly massive number of people from around the world. All I can do is relate to you my experiences and the experiences of hundreds of thousands of people and hope that it will intrigue you sufficiently to at least try it for ten days and see for yourself.

There are a couple more points I wish to make before bringing this chapter to a close. Regardless of what you think about what I've written here about fruit, please just view what I am going to say from a strictly commonsense perspective.

Do you know what group can be relied upon most consistently to give an honest and accurate appraisal of fruit? Children. Little kids haven't been indoctrinated and propagandized by special interests into taking sides based on a bunch of statistics and opinions. No, little kids react from their instincts and emotions. Go to the grocery store and just watch little children react as soon as they catch sight of fruit. "Mommy, mommy, I want some cherries!" "Ooh, watermelon! Can we have some watermelon?" "Please, please, let's get strawberries!" They can hardly be contained.

There are rural areas in practically every state in the United States where the public can walk into orchards and onto farms and pick their own fruit: blueberries, strawberries, blackberries, apples. Ask kids if they want to go pick their own berries and watch their reaction. It's always the same thing: their faces light up as though Christmas came early. Why is that? Why do you think children *always* have such an immediate, heartfelt, positive reaction to the prospect of picking and eating their own fruit? An innocent, unaffected child can always be trusted to give an earnest and honest appraisal. Place a slab of cooked liver and a bowl of fruit in front of a kid and see which s/he reaches for. It's no contest.

Throughout the world there are thousands of different varieties of fruit. The very first and most important line of defense that we humans have to protect ourselves against anything harmful entering our bodies is our senses. Is fruit not a veritable celebration for the senses? If something looks repulsive, would you be inclined to eat it? If something smells foul, would you be tempted to put it in your mouth? If something tastes nasty, would you chew it up and swallow it? Fruit is the exact opposite of this. It is inviting to our senses in every way.

Is there anything quite as aromatic and enticing as the sweet scent of a fully ripe peach? Can anything surpass the luscious flavor of a fresh-cut slice of watermelon on a hot day? And, of course, fruit is a feast for the eyes. Can any artist's pallet rival the spectacular circus of colors that a table laden with a wide variety of fruit can? Fruit looks, smells, and tastes as good as anything that can be put into the body.

Does it make sense to you that the Grand Creator would blanket the earth with every beautifully colored, pleasantly scented, and delectable tasting fruit imaginable only to play a monstrous trick on us—that is, to intentionally entice us with fruit so that we will eat it and become sick? Only someone completely devoid of the physiological and biological needs of the living body and lacking any vestige of common sense would suggest such a completely bizarre and illogical notion as that.

The reason why fruit is supremely pleasing to our senses is to assure us that it is a perfect food perfectly suited for the human diet. And when eaten *correctly, it will do more good than any other food you eat.*

6

You Gotta Move!
Exercising For Fat Loss

Writing a book about diet and weight loss and not mentioning the role of exercise would be a little like writing a book about our solar system and leaving out the name of one of the planets. I have no intention of belaboring the point; it is highly unlikely that you are not already well aware of the importance of exercise, so one more critique of the statistics proving that to be so certainly isn't going to make a difference. I do think I have a few interesting tidbits to share however.

Before going one word further, on the outside chance you skip this chapter altogether or give it only short shrift, I *must* share with you the number-one reason why some form of exercise is beyond crucial, not only to your effort to lose weight but also to your health and longevity. I think I made the point well earlier in the book about what an extraordinary gift and amazing mechanism the lymph system is. Without an efficiently functioning lymph system no health goal is reachable.

The human bloodstream is sometimes referred to as "the river of life" because it is responsible for bringing oxygenated blood to every cell of the body, without which we would quickly perish. At the center of the remarkable cardiovascular system is the heart, serving as the pump to see to it that the bloodstream is always flowing. Lymph fluid must always be flowing in the body as well, but it has no pumping mechanism as the cardiovascular system does. Instead, it is entirely dependent upon physical activity—exercise! Learning this particular bit of physiological truth sure does put the need for physical activity in a whole new light, doesn't it? Depriving your body of physical exercise is in effect impeding the activities of your lymph system and *asking* for problems—you might just as well get down on your knees and pray for some type of health challenge. And *that* prayer, I assure you, *will* be answered.

It isn't only an inferior diet that causes excess body fat to be stored; an equal contributor is lack of activity. Just look at the structure of the living body—it's made for movement! To a very large extent, the reason why diets regularly fail is because of insufficient exercise. A sluggish metabolism is not the ally of someone wishing to lose weight. Increasing physical activity speeds up metabolism and that translates into more fat loss. I just wish to briefly touch on two extremely simple, yet highly effective, methods of exercise—either one of which, or both, will surely help optimize weight loss right along with the dietary suggestions I've made and taking Slender GR™.

AEROBIC EXERCISE

The first is aerobic exercise, or what is referred to as "cardio." Increasing the amount of aerobic exercise you do will definitely increase your metabolic rate *and* burn fat. The literal meaning of the word "aerobic" is "with oxygen" or "in the presence of oxygen." Fat will only be burned as fuel in the presence of oxygen. The longer the duration of aerobic exercise, the more oxygen there is, and the more fat burning will occur. That's because stored glycogen is used up first; but once it's burned up, the body goes for the fat for fuel.

There are so many aerobic exercises to choose from, there's bound to be something that appeals to you: walking, jogging, bicycling, swimming, volleyball, tennis—the list goes on and on.

Walk Those Pounds Away!

In terms of a highly effective aerobic exercise that can be moderate and unstructured and still be highly beneficial, walking is ideal. Walking oxygenates the blood, which in turn supplies oxygen to all your cells; it helps increase the strength and efficiency of your heart and muscles; it lowers cholesterol (the kind you don't want); and it even reduces high blood pressure.

There is an artificial growth hormone administered to people over sixty to help reduce fat. It is expensive and it has serious side effects. Walking as little as twenty minutes a day has been shown to stimulate the production of this hormone. Walking also can be instrumental in helping you lose weight; a 45 minute walk every other day for a year can burn 18 pounds of fat. Mile for mile, walking is actually a better fat burner than running; walking four miles burns more fat than running the same distance in less time. And, of course, walking stimulates the lymph system. Walking is a winner!

Bounce for Life!—The Benefits of Rebounding

I'll tell you what I think one of the very best all-around aerobic exercises is, and it is something I do every day without fail: rebounding. Rebounding has been around since 1936 and is used by world-class athletes. You can purchase a rebounder-or "mini-trampoline" as they are frequently called— very inexpensively, and put it anywhere in your home for convenient use. Rebounding couldn't be easier. Not only is it a great aerobic exercise but it also avoids the joint-jarring shock to the knees, ankles, and lower back that jogging and running on a hard surface do.

For me, the most important aspect of rebounding is the phenomenal impact it has on the lymph system. All it calls for is a slight up-and-down bounce, which need be only three or four inches to reap benefit, but can be higher. The higher the jump the more intense the workout and the better the overall results. The alternating weightlessness and increased gravitational pull subjects the body to a change in velocity and direction with each bounce. At the bottom of the bounce, all the literally millions of one-way valves of the lymph system are closed because of the pressure above them. At the top of the bounce, the valves are open, allowing the lymph fluid to flow up as the body starts down. Every valve opens at the same time, allowing and stimulating the flow of lymph fluid. As little or as much rebounding as you do can be of tremendous benefit to the lymph system. And its benefits are cumulative! If you bounce up and down on your rebounder for three minutes ten times during the day, it is the same benefit as rebounding for 30 minutes straight once a day!

You can also do more than just bouncing on the rebounder in order to increase the positive effects. You can do jumping jacks with each bounce, which will really get your heart beating. Also, you can use weights while bouncing. I am talking about very light, handheld weights, only one or perhaps two pounds. As you bounce you hold the weights by your thighs and curl your arms so your hands come up near your shoulders. This gives you a very good workout.

There are so many benefits to rebounding I can't list them all, but it affects nearly every organ and system in the body; it even helps stimulate metabolism. NASA has studied the effects of rebounding and has found it to be superior to walking, running, or treadmills as a means of effective exercise. In space, astronauts tend to lose bone mass because of weightlessness. During training, NASA utilizes rebound exercise and has found it increases bone density. You need only search "benefits of rebounding" online to see how extensively this one exercise positively contributes to your health and well-being. The person who put rebounding "on the map" was Albert E. Carter, and his book *The Miracle of Rebound Exercise* is still considered to be the bible of rebounding.

If you commit to doing some type of aerobic exercise, it would be best to get in the habit of doing so during the morning hours. When you awaken in the morning you have essentially been fasting for eight hours or so. That means your body's storehouse of glycogen is low, which causes more fat to be burned. Also, there is less actual glucose in the blood, which also causes more fat to be burned.

In addition to morning aerobic exercise waking you up and energizing you, there are some psychological advantages. By exercising in the morning, you start the day with a feeling of accomplishment that lasts all day—instead of worrying all day that you haven't exercised yet. Besides, you know how it is, you keep putting exercise off until later, and something else comes up that takes precedence, and all of a sudden the day's over or you're too tired, and it doesn't get done at all. Better to do it in the morning and feel good about yourself.

There was actually a study conducted in 1990 on this very subject to see what time of day exercise is done with most regularity. It revealed that when exercise is performed during the morning hours 75 percent stuck with it, while 75 percent of those who exercised at any other time of day dropped their exercise regimen.

WEIGHT TRAINING

There is a second way to lose fat with exercise and that is by weight training. Let me tell you right at the start, I am no expert on weight training to lose weight, not even close. So I am not going to be recommending some particular regimen. Rather, I suggest that if your interest is piqued, you seek out someone to help you who is knowledgeable on the subject. I am bringing it up because I know that it can be useful. I think when the average person thinks of weight lifting or bodybuilding they automatically think that it is a way to put *on* weight, but the fact is, if done in a very specific way, it can also result in taking off weight.

Ask any bodybuilder and he or she will tell you that muscles are their best friend in losing fat because muscles are like a furnace, a metabolic furnace, when it comes to burning fat. The more muscle on the body, the more fat is burned—even while you are sleeping! But rather than lifting heavy weights, weight training involves using very light to moderate weights and doing more repetitions and sets. And when properly done and combined with aerobic exercise, it can be a very powerful weight-losing strategy. So, it's something you can think about investigating. But at the very least, do some walking or get a rebounder—or both! You gotta move!

7

INTERVIEW WITH DR. MAMADOU ON ENZYMES

Dr. M. Mamadou is currently the chief scientific officer of Phytomedic Labs, LLC. He has taught and conducted research at several universities and has provided consulting and research services for many health- and nutrition-related companies. His scientific interests include disease prevention, nutritional disorders, degenerative diseases, enzymology (the study of enzymes), and food sciences and technology. Actively involved in enzyme-based formulations for health and wellness, his present research interest focuses on isolating new phytochemicals and enzymes for health and wellness dietary supplements as well as lecturing all over the world on nutrition and wellness. Dr. Mamadou was kind enough to provide the answers to some frequently asked questions about enzymes.

●●●● What are enzymes?

DR. MAMADOU: Enzymes are unique proteins that act as catalysts in helping the body perform the trillions of biochemical reactions necessary to sustain life, which take place every minute within the 75 to 100 trillion cells of the body. They primarily speed up biochemical reactions. What this means is that without enzymes, the reactions necessary for life would not occur fast enough for it to be sustained.

A good example of this is how enzymes support the digestive process. It would be impossible to digest food without the enzymes that are naturally a part of the digestive system. Enzymes are secreted in the mouth, the stomach, and the intestinal tract. They break down or digest proteins, fats, and carbohydrates. Though we can grind these foods down into smaller pieces with our teeth and swallow the food, we would not be able to benefit from the nutrients in the foods without these vital, active proteins.

●●●● *Are there different types of enzymes?*

DR. MAMADOU: This is a bit of a tricky question. Some scientists would answer this by describing enzymes that break down molecules, enzymes that put molecules together, enzymes that build molecules, and finally enzymes that change the structure or function of a molecule.

Really though, what is most important to understand when it comes to enzymes and nutrition is that they can be differentiated in several ways. The types of food they digest, their source, and their primary application are what differentiate enzymes.

By type of food:

❏ Proteases (also called proteolytic enzymes, proteinases, peptidases) digest proteins

❏ Lipase digests fats

❏ Amylases (sometimes called carbohydrases) digest starch

By source:

❏ Animal based (pancreatin, trypsin, chymotrypsin)

❏ Plant-based or fungal (amylase, lipase and protease)

❏ Bacterial (nattokinase, serrapeptase)

❏ Plant (bromelain and papain)

By application:

❏ Therapeutic

❏ Digestive

●●●● *Why are enzymes important to overall health?*

DR. MAMADOU: To answer that, I would like to first talk about two important aspects of health and wellness. The first is nutrition; every living organism including humans requires the proper nutrients to maintain life, to reproduce, to help fight disease—basically to survive. At the core of good and healthy living is the ability to consume and absorb these nutrients at the cellular level. The immune system, for example, cannot protect us from harm when we are not adequately providing the immune cells with the essential nutrients they need.

The second important aspect consists of the timely delivery of nutrients, immune molecules, and so on, as well as the timely elimination of metabolic wastes. The delivery and elimination are primarily preformed by the circulatory system and the lymph system. The blood and lymph systems make up the transport system within the body and when this transport system is impaired it has severe negative consequences to all other key systems of the body.

❑ Nutrients are not delivered properly and on time.

❑ Adequate oxygen supply to the cells is compromised.

❑ Adequate carbon dioxide removal from the tissues is ineffective.

❑ The immune system cannot efficiently perform its protective functions.

❑ Hormone production decreases.

The interesting thing about this, though, is that the keys to overall health; proper nutrition, supply of nutrients, and elimination, are absolutely dependent upon enzymes. The demand placed on the body to keep up with the needs required to supply nutrients to the cells and properly eliminate toxins is enormous. Considering the poor food sources, environmental challenges, external stresses, poor sleeping habits, and the like that we are exposed to on a daily basis, it is important to support the body with enzymes. In effect, as we age we cannot meet the demand we have created. It is because of this that I always recommend supplemental digestive enzymes.

●●●● *How do enzymes assist in weight loss?*

DR. MAMADOU: The action of dietary supplemental enzymes is very important to weight management and weight loss. For instance, efficiently digesting foods with the help of supplemental enzymes ensures that the body receives the nutrients it needs in a timely manner. When foods are not properly digested and nutrients assimilated, the body sends food-craving signals leading to higher calorie intake. This cycle leads to weight gain and can also contribute to eating disorders. When nutrients are properly supplied, the signals sent tell the body it has what it needs and hunger dissipates.

Additionally, supplemental digestive enzymes improve and maintain good circulation. Poor circulation, characterized by inefficient oxygen supply and removal of carbon dioxide, causes constant fatigue, thus increasing the risk for weight gain. Enzymes could also help in weight management by promoting the breakdown of fats in the body (lipolysis).

Finally, a special enzyme blend called Glucoreductase™, which can be found in the Enzymedica product Slender GR, can convert simple sugars into fiber. This has two very beneficial results when it comes to weight management and weight loss. First, it helps balance blood sugar and as a result balances insulin demand (insulin is a hormone that balances blood sugar). When insulin demand is high it forces the body to store fat, by reducing this demand the body begins to burn fat as a metabolic energy source. Additionally, this enzyme blend has the ability to reduce the caloric value of foods. Approximately 30 percent of the starchy carbohydrates that are so often blamed for adding inches to the waistline can be converted to fiber that serves as a food source for the microflora of the intestinal tract. This conversion prevents these calories from turning to fat. Please see the Appendix with Dr. Steven Lamm for more information.

●●●● *Can I get the enzymes I need from the food I eat?*

DR. MAMADOU: Though enzymes are present in fresh, raw foods, these enzymes do little to satisfy the needs of the body. Let's consider a hard, unripe banana. If it is left for a few days, it starts softening. Over time it becomes ripe. This transformation is due to the enzymes present in the banana, which break down its starch into simple sugars. However, the enzymes that convert an unsweetened, hard unripe banana into a sweet one are not available to benefit the digestive process in the gut. There are not surplus enzymes contained in raw foods beyond what is needed to digest each particular food. Nature provides enough enzymes to support the digestion of the food in which they are present, but there would be none left over to provide additional support for anything else.

●●●● *How and when should I take enzymes?*

DR. MAMADOU: Supplemental digestive enzymes, including the weight-loss enzyme blend found in Slender GR™, should be taken with meals to optimize the digestive process and alleviate gastric discomfort. They can also be taken during less active times of the digestive process (often referred to as "in-between meals") to provide a systemic benefit such as would help control inflammation or enhance circulation

When taking enzymes with meals, it is best to take them at the beginning of the meal, usually with the first bite of food. This allows a good mixing of the enzymes with the meal and ensures that the enzymes have sufficient access to the variety of food molecules contained in a typical meal. If a person happens to forget to take their enzymes at the beginning of the meal, I tell them to do so as soon as they remember. The truth is, the body is in a constant state of digestion and enzymes can support that process at any time, so it is better to take them as soon as you remember then to not take them at all.

●●●● *What is the source of enzymes?*

DR. MAMADOU: The sources are described in different ways when enzymes are used for supplemental purposes. They are primarily described as animal, plant and plant-based, though technically the "plant-based" would likely be described in a lab setting as fungal or microbial.

Early enzyme therapy studies were done using animal-derived enzymes that originate from the pancreas of a pig. Although these enzymes are helpful, they do not survive stomach acid. As a result of this deficiency, animal enzymes must be protected by enteric coating. This chemical coating allows the enzyme to pass through the stomach and into the small intestine without being denatured. I should also add that there have been recent concerns regarding animal diseases that could be transmitted to humans. This has slowed down the production and commercialization of pancreatic enzymes as dietary supplements.

The most popular source of supplemental enzymes is plant-based. Plant-based enzymes should not be confused with plant-derived enzymes such as bromelain and papain from pineapple and papaya. Plant-based enzymes are actually enzymes that are derived from non-harmful fungus and bacteria and are known for their wide pH range of alkalinity and acidity. This unique trait provides a tremendous benefit since they will work in the various compartments of the gastrointestinal tract and are active and stable in the gastric environment of the stomach. In my opinion, they are the most suitable as dietary supplements for health and wellness.

I would like to add that since enzymes are derived from various organisms, it is important to look for a well-known, reputable provider of enzyme supplements. There are excellent enzyme suppliers and dietary supplement manufacturers that exercise due diligence in their production, purification, and handling to ensure that high-quality, pure, and effective enzymes are available to the consumer.

● ● ● ● *Is there a benefit to how enzymes are blended?*

DR. MAMADOU: Yes, there are numerous benefits to blending enzymes. Let's use protease as an example. I mentioned earlier that proteases are the enzymes that break down proteins; what I have not explained is that enzymes are very specific and so one protease cannot break down all the proteins we regularly consume in our diet. To overcome this inherent challenge, I recommend that formulators blend various proteases in a manner that their actions could complement each other in order to completely breakdown these proteins. In fact, the blending of all enzymes in nutritional supplement formulas is crucial in determining the quality of various enzyme products on the market. A good example of this is the enzyme blend Glucoreductase™ found in the product Slender GR™. It contains several enzymes, which include transglucosidase, lipase and protease. Each of these ingredients, though beneficial are unlikely to have a profound effect on weight-loss or blood sugar, yet as a blend have been proven to be very beneficial for both.

● ● ● ● *Can enzymes help with other health issues?*

DR. MAMADOU: I am so glad I am getting a chance to talk briefly about this. The fact is, enzymes help with so many things it's hard to know where to begin. Supplemental enzymes can have a beneficial effect on numerous systems of the body; this is why they are often called systemic enzymes. In particular, the proteolytic enzymes, or proteases, have been shown to be absorbed into the blood after being consumed orally. The beneficial actions of these enzymes alone include:

❑ Preventing attachment of bacteria to tissue thereby reducing or eliminating risk.

❑ Acting as adjunct to cancer therapies: studies have shown that supplemental enzymes help control some tumor cell growth and metastasis.

❑ Helping prevent clogging of blood vessels by fibrin and thrombocytes.

❑ Controlling inflammatory processes, thus limiting the onset of chronic inflammations.

❑ Enhancing blood flow to help deliver hormones and immune cells, and remove metabolic wastes.

• • •

As supplemental enzymes promote good circulation, they help provide energy, which promotes physical exercise. This is obviously an important factor in weight management and weight-loss programs.

8

RECIPES FOR LIFE

GOOD AND GOOD FOR YOU

Natalia KW, Contributor

YUMMM ... THE FOOD SECTION. Now we're talkin'. This chapter presents, for your continued weight-loss success and maintenance, a variety of lip-smacking, living-food recipes. At first I considered including some healthy cooked recipes for some variety, but let's face it, there is no shortage of recipes for cooked food. You could practically close your eyes and hurl a stone in any direction and it would land on a recipe for something cooked.

And for those of you laboring under the false impression that all there can be to living foods are salads and anything else would be like eating cardboard and tree bark, you are in for a very pleasant surprise. I have eaten meals consisting of only living food that, tastewise and presentation-wise, would rival any meal of cooked foods and would delight and stun the palate of even the most highly sophisticated chef.

One of the most highly accomplished and well-respected living food proponents and chefs I know is author Natalia KW, well known for her scrumptious, innovative gustatory creations. It would not be at all surprising to hear someone say, after tasting one of Natalia's dishes, something to the effect of, "Are you trying to tell me that something this delicious is actually *good* for me?" I am *so* pleased to say that Natalia has most graciously agreed to provide the recipes for this book. You are in for a real treat if the pleasure and variety of living food is something relatively new to you. I could go on talking about Natalia's accomplishments and the transformation that took place in her life as a result of living foods, but I will let her introduce herself, and her recipes, to you. This is what Natalia KW has to say:

"My passion for living food runs deep. I have seen a dramatic trans-formation in my life and in the lives of those around me when incorpo-rating a healthy amount of fresh, raw, and organic plant foods. In a world where we have been barely surviving on processed foods, devoid of nutrition, our bodies awaken when they begin to be treated properly. True nourishment from the rich nutrient profiles of living foods gifts us with increased energy and immunity, allows our body to detoxify and assists us with natural weight loss. From losing excess pounds to miracu-lously healing deadly diseases, the living food diet brings forth an impressive number of testimonials for all around life improvement.

In my own life, there was a time when, as a young woman, I was overly medicated and truly ill. From excessive antibiotic use, my entire body was overrun with Candida, and I was constantly run down, exhausted, and sick. I ran from practitioner to practitioner, looking to buy the latest "cure," but continued to find myself frustrated and defeated. One fateful day, my brother recommended living foods as a way to boost my immunity and heal my imbalances. I was instantly inspired, knowing that it was time for me to heal from within. After a few months of cleansing and detoxification on a 100-percent living food diet, I found my body was able to correct the imbalance all on its own. With the proper fuel and nourishment, I was feeling better than I had in years. The transformation in my life has been radical. My immune system is rock solid—even things like the "common" cold are a distant memory. Becoming nourished, and healing on such a deep level, has brought a massive amount of joy into my life and has allowed me to reach goal after goal. After experiencing such a profound and joyful rebirth, I knew that I had to make it my life's mission to share this information with others, so that they too could experience such a high quality of life.

I have worked with restaurants and private clients, from people that were "just curious" to those with life threatening diseases. What I have found to be true in many cases is that as impressive as the benefits of living foods are, many people feel overwhelmed with the idea of such a dramatic lifestyle change. What is so important to keep in mind is that this is never a game of all or nothing; the more living, fresh plant foods that you can incorporate into your daily life, the better. It's as simple as that—add more living foods, experience the benefits, and with those benefits in mind, continue down the path to your ultimate well-being.

I have been on the standard American diet, a vegetarian diet, a vegan diet, allergen-free diets . . . the list goes on. I have seen extreme deprivation in my life and have felt deficient and malnourished, even while consuming large amounts of food. Nothing compares to the joy I have felt from the true nourishment of pure, living foods. One of the biggest factors of being deeply nourished for me is that these foods must taste absolutely divine. Since 2007, I have spent countless hours in the kitchen experimenting with recipes, constantly challenging myself to create the most delicious living food recipes on the planet. At the same time, my rule is to always make these recipes accessible to all, using readily available ingredients and techniques. The result is a library of luscious recipes that even a newcomer can whip up and enjoy tonight. From my cookbook, Pure Pleasures, *to the recipes shared here, my ultimate goal is to offer you dishes that not only assist you in your effort to lose weight, but also satisfy, nourish and heal on a complete body, mind, and spirit level.*

From simple smoothies and salads to delectable entrees and desserts, I encourage you to have fun creating these new recipes. Watch as your palate expands and your cravings shift when your body experiences the pleasure of pure foods. If at any moment you are feeling the slightest bit deprived, create one of my dessert recipes and watch that feeling disappear. Your success with living foods for the long term will rely on your enjoyment of them, making this a habit you want to stick with. I wish for you to enjoy my recipes in the best of health and happiness and when you're hungry for more, please visit my website, www.NataliaKW.com for even more inspiration."

BEVERAGES
&
BREAKFASTS

SWEET LIME
GREEN JUICE

*Starting your day with fresh green juice gives
you instant revitalization. This juice is sweet,
tangy, and very refreshing.*

Serves 2

4 green apples, cored

2 large cucumbers

1/2 bunch spinach

1 handful mint

1 lime, with skin

Run all ingredients through your juicer. Serve and enjoy!

REJUVENATION JUICE

Great any time of day—so refreshing!

Serves 2

• •

5 or 6 apples

6–8 stalks of celery

Core the apples to remove the seeds. Run all ingredients through your juicer. For best taste, the mix should be approximately three-quarters apple juice and one-quarter celery juice.

● ● ●

MORNING SUNSHINE SMOOTHIE

This is a particularly simple but tasty blend.
It is one that kids seem to really like.

Serves 2

• •

2 cups fresh orange juice

1 banana
(frozen or not—if frozen,
smoothie will be thicker*)

1/2 cup frozen strawberries

1/2 cup frozen blueberries

Place all ingredients in a blender and blend until very smooth. Serve.

* To freeze bananas, peel, break into pieces, and place in airtight container.

CHERRY VANILLA CREAM SMOOTHIE

*After a good night's sleep, you want to ease your body back
into digestion, and blended smoothies are the perfect way to do this.
Plus, this will keep you satisfied until lunch!*

Serves 2

. . . .

2 cups pure water

1/2 cup raw cashews

2 tablespoons raw honey

1 vanilla bean or 1/2 teaspoon of vanilla extract

2 cups frozen cherries

1 frozen banana

Place the water, cashews, honey, and vanilla in a high-speed
blender and blend until smooth and creamy. Add the cherries
and the banana, and blend again until frosty.

TROPICAL GREEN SMOOTHIE

*Green smoothies are a living-food favorite.
Nutritious greens hide behind the sweetness of luscious fruits,
giving you a huge early morning health boost. The coconut oil in
this smoothie adds richness to keep you full and nourished.*

Serves 2

. . . .

1 cup pure water

2 cups kale

1 cup chopped pineapple

1 cup chopped mango

2 tablespoons cold-pressed coconut oil*

2 frozen bananas

In a blender, blend water, kale, pineapple, mango, and coconut oil until very smooth. Add the frozen bananas and blend again until thick and frosty. Serve and enjoy.

*Visit http://nutiva.com/products/10_coconut.php

CHOCOLATE-MINT-SPIRULINA SMOOTHIE

*Spirulina is another way to turn your smoothie green.
It is blue-green algae in powder form that is full of vitamins
and minerals and boasts a 60-percent protein content.
It nicely complements raw chocolate, and with a hint of mint,
this is like having dessert for breakfast.*

Serves 2

1 1/2 cups pure water

1/4 cup raw macadamia nuts

2 tablespoons raw honey

3 ripe bananas

2 tablespoons raw cacao powder

1 tablespoon spirulina (or green powder of your choice)

1/8 teaspoon organic peppermint extract

Place the water, macadamia nuts, and honey in a high-speed blender and blend until smooth. Add the bananas, cacao, spirulina, and peppermint and blend again to combine. Serve and enjoy!

PINEAPPLE-GOJI-CHIA PUDDING

In the living food world, we liken chia seeds to tapioca. This makes a rich, creamy, filling breakfast and is an excellent food for digestive health.

Serves 4

• •

2 cups water

1/3 cup raw cashews

4–6 pitted Medjool dates

1 vanilla bean or 1/2 teaspoon vanilla extract

pinch of Himalayan salt

5–6 tablespoons chia seeds

1 1/2 cups fresh pineapple, chopped

1/3 cup goji berries (or raisins)

1/4 cup shredded coconut

In a high-speed blender combine the water, cashews, dates, vanilla, and salt. Blend until smooth. Pour into a bowl and whisk in the chia seeds. Begin with 5 tablespoons. Let stand for 10 minutes to thicken. Stir to break up any clumps and add an additional tablespoon of chia seeds if you desire a thicker pudding. When it's to your liking, stir in the pineapple and goji berries. Sprinkle with shredded coconut and serve.

● ● ●

SUPER TRAIL MIX BARS

When you need breakfast or a snack on the go, making your own portable bars is perfect! These are very satisfying and of course, tasty.

Makes 10 bars

• •

2 cups raw cashews

3/4 cup pitted Medjool dates

1/3 cup raw honey

1 cup shredded coconut

1/4 teaspoon vanilla extract

pinch of Himalayan salt

1/4 cup dried cranberries

1/4 cup raw cacao nibs

1/4 cup hemp seeds*

Place the cashews in your food processor fit with the S-blade. Process until finely ground. Add the dates, honey, coconut, vanilla, and salt and process again to combine. Finally add the cranberries, cacao nibs, and hemp seeds, and pulse gently just to distribute these ingredients evenly. Press into a 9-inch square pan. Cut into ten equal bars. Wrap individually in parchment paper for a grab-and-go snack.

*Visit https://store.nutiva.com/hempseed/

● ● ● ●

APPLE RAISIN GRANOLA WITH VANILLA CASHEW MILK

This is a very hearty breakfast, perfect for weekends when you're craving something extra special.

Serves 2

Granola

1 cup raw Brazil Nuts

2 teaspoons cinnamon

1/8 teaspoon nutmeg

1/2 teaspoon fresh ginger

pinch of Himalayan salt

2 small apples,
cored and roughly chopped

2 tablespoons raw honey

1/4 cup raisins

Place the Brazil nuts, cinnamon, nutmeg, ginger ,and salt in your food processor fit with the S-blade. Pulse to chop. Add the apples and honey and pulse again to combine. Do not overprocess; you do want some texture to remain. Stir the raisins in by hand. Divide into two bowls.

● ● ●

VANILLA CASHEW MILK

*This is a wonderfully delicious and nutritious
alternative to milk.
Great on fruit salads also.*

Serves 2

● ●

1 1/4 cups water

1/3 cup raw cashews

2 tablespoons honey

1/2 teaspoon vanilla extract

Place all ingredients in a high-speed blender and blend until very smooth. Pour over the granola and serve. Store any remaining milk in the refrigerator.

DIPS & DRESSINGS

CREAMY PESTO

This is a lighter version of a traditional pesto—nut, oil, and dairy free, but still rich with flavor.

Serves 2

1 ripe Hass avocado

4 ounces fresh basil leaves

2 cloves of garlic

2 teaspoons lemon juice

3/4 teaspoon Himalayan salt

Place the garlic in the food processor and process until finely chopped. Cut the avocado in half and remove the pit and the skin. Place in the food processor. Add the lemon and process until creamy. Add in the basil and salt and process again until well combined. Serve over zucchini noodles or on top of thick tomato slices and enjoy!

RED PEPPER HUMMUS

This is a living food twist on a Mediterranean favorite, replacing cooked chickpeas with sprouted sunflower seeds. This is very hearty and super satisfying on top of green salads or with cucumber slices for dipping.

Serves 6–8

• •

4 cloves of garlic

1 1/2 cups raw sunflower seeds, soaked for 4-6 hours, drained and rinsed

1/2 cup raw sesame tahini

1 red bell pepper, seeded and roughly chopped

1/2 cup fresh lemon juice

6 tablespoons cold-pressed olive oil

2 teaspoons paprika

1 teaspoon Himalayan salt

Place the garlic in a food processor and pulse to chop. Add all remaining ingredients to the food processor and process very well until you achieve a smooth and thick consistency, which may take a few minutes. Serve over greens or with vegetable slices for dipping.

● ● ●

CREAMY CUCUMBER DILL DIP

Creamy and fresh with a little bit of cucumber crunch, this flavorful dip is great with carrots and bell peppers or wrapped up in lettuce leaves and topped with sprouts.

Serves 2

• •

1 ripe Hass avocado

3/4 cup diced cucumber

2 tablespoons fresh dill, chopped

juice of 1/2 lemon

1/2 teaspoon Himalayan salt

1 clove garlic, minced

1 tablespoon diced sweet onion

Place the avocado in a bowl and mash well with a fork. Add in all remaining ingredients and mix well. Serve with vegetables for dipping or wrapping.

● ● ●

PARSLEY GARLIC CREAM

This is a delicious, zesty green dip, perfect for crudités.

Serves 6–8

1 cup raw cashews,
soaked 3 hours,
drained and rinsed

1 bunch fresh parsley

1/4 cup hemp seed

1/2 cup pure water

1/4 cup lemon juice

1/4 cup olive oil

3 cloves of garlic

3/4 teaspoon Himalayan salt

1/8 teaspoon cayenne pepper

Place all ingredients in a high-speed blender and blend until very smooth. Serve chilled.

FRESH SALADS

EMERALD KALE SALAD

*Kale salads are delicious beyond your wildest expectations!
Join the club of kale lovers! With a little culinary magic,
salt will transform the tough leaves into tender green ribbons,
ready to absorb a flavorful marinade. This salad is jazzed up
with dill, pumpkin seeds, and avocado—yum!*

Serves 2

1 bunch Lacinato kale

1/4 – 1/2 teaspoon Himalayan salt

1 clove of garlic, minced

3 tablespoons olive oil

2 tablespoons fresh lemon juice

2 tablespoon chopped dill

3 tablespoons raw pumpkin seeds

1/2 cup halved cherry tomatoes

1/2 avocado, chopped into half-inch pieces

2 tablespoons diced red onion

Freshly ground black pepper to taste

Wash kale and remove the stems. Stacking several leaves at a time, cut the kale into thin strips. Place the kale in a large bowl and sprinkle with the salt. Massage the kale with your hands for several minutes until it begins to soften and wilt. Add the olive oil, lemon, and garlic and continue to massage. Toss in the remaining ingredients and mix well.

SESAME GINGER CRUNCH

This salad packs a satisfying crunch and the vegetables are perfectly complemented by a flavorful, Asian inspired dressing.

Serves 4

* *

CRUNCHY SALAD

2¹/2 cups shredded cabbage

1 cup shredded carrot

¹/2 cup bean sprouts

¹/2 cup diced red bell pepper

¹/2 cup chopped broccoli florets

¹/2 cup pea pods

¹/4 cup chopped cilantro leaves

¹/4 cup chopped scallions

¹/2 cup raw cashews

2 tablespoons black sesame seeds

Toss all ingredients in a large bowl.

SESAME GINGER DRESSING

³/4 cup cold pressed sesame oil

¹/4 cup coconut aminos, Nama Shoyu, or wheat-free tamari

2 tablespoons raw honey

2 cloves of garlic, minced

1 teaspoon grated ginger

¹/2 teaspoon lime zest

¹/4 teaspoon crushed chili pepper

Whisk all ingredients together in a medium bowl until well combined. Pour over salad and toss well. Taste for salt and add a pinch if necessary.

CILANTRO LIME
COLE SLAW

This is a zesty take on a
classic picnic salad,
full of crunch, flavor, and color.

Serves 4–6

. . . .

COLE SLAW

5 cups finely shredded cabbage

1 1/2 cups shredded carrot

1 cup red bell pepper, julienned

1/2 cup red onion,
cut into very thin strips

Toss all ingredients in a large bowl.

CILANTRO-LIME MAYO

1/2 cup pure water

1/3 cup fresh lime juice

1 1/2 cups raw pine nuts
or cashews

2 cloves of garlic

1 teaspoon ground chipotle pepper

3/4 teaspoon Himalayan salt

1/2 cup chopped cilantro leaves

Place the water, lime juice, pine nuts or cashews, garlic, chipotle, and salt in a high-speed blender and blend until very smooth. Fold in the cilantro by hand. Pour over the cole slaw and mix very well.

MEDITERRANEAN SALAD

*In my world, nothing beats a garden fresh,
green salad. This makes a nourishing meal when
topped with my red pepper hummus.*

Serves 4

. . . .

SALAD

1 head romaine lettuce,
washed and chopped

1 cup sliced cucumber

1 cup diced tomatoes

1/2 cup diced red bell pepper

1/3 cup diced sweet onion

1/3 cup chopped sun dried black olives

Toss all ingredients in a large bowl.

LEMON THYME DRESSING

1/2 cup fresh lemon juice

3 cloves of garlic

2 tablespoons sweet onion

1 teaspoon Himalayan salt

1/2 teaspoon black pepper

2/3 cup cold-pressed olive oil

1 tablespoon fresh thyme leaves

Blend together the lemon juice, garlic, onion, salt, and pepper.
Slowly add the olive oil while blending to emulsify. Lastly, add
the thyme leaves and blend very gently just to combine and
release the flavors. Pour over the salad and toss well.

TOMATO BASIL SALAD

*This is perfect for a hot summer day when
tomatoes are at their peak of ripeness.*

Serves 2

. . . .

2 large heirloom tomatoes, diced

1/2 cup fresh basil leaves, roughly chopped

2 scallions, finely chopped

2 cloves of garlic, minced

2 tablespoons cold-pressed olive oil

1/4 teaspoon Himalayan salt

pinch of black pepper, to taste

1/4 cup raw pine nuts

Toss all ingredients except for the pine nuts in a medium
bowl. Divide the salad among two bowls and sprinkle with
pine nuts when serving.

NOURISHING ENTREES

FARMER'S MARKET WRAPS WITH RED PEPPER "CHEESE"

Get to know your local organic farmer! You can have fun experimenting with this recipe according to the fresh veggies you can find in season. The red pepper cheese makes this dish ultra tasty.

Serves 4

● ●

WRAPS

4 large collard leaves

3 cups chopped lettuce

1 cup shredded carrots

1 large tomato, diced

1/2 cup diced cucumber

1/2 bell pepper, cut into strips

1/2 cup sunflower sprouts

1/4 cup fresh parsley, chopped

3 tablespoons olive oil

2 teaspoons lemon juice

1/4 teaspoon salt

black pepper to taste

Wash your collard leaves and trim the thick stem. In a large bowl, toss together the lettuce, carrots, tomato, cucumber, bell pepper, sprouts, and parsley. If you are going to eat the wraps right away, toss with the olive oil, lemon, salt, and pepper. Otherwise, wait until serving as the vegetables will wilt.

RED PEPPER CHEESE

1 cup raw cashews

1/2 cup chopped red bell pepper

2 tablespoons lemon juice

1/4 cup water

1 small garlic clove

1/2 teaspoon paprika

1/2 teaspoon oregano

1/4 teaspoon miso

1/4 teaspoon Himalayan salt

Place all ingredients in a high-speed blender and blend well until smooth and creamy.

To assemble: Place a collard leaf flat on cutting board. Spread 1/4 cup of red pepper cheese onto each leaf. Top with 1/4 of the veggies and roll up. Continue with each leaf until all of the collards and veggies are used.

● ● ●

COCONUT CAULIFLOWER RICE WITH MANGO SALSA

*Living food is all about getting ultra creative with your veggies.
Here artfully chopped cauliflower and finely shredded coconut
will take the place of traditional rice. With a hint of lime,
a sprinkle of cilantro and a topping of juicy mango salsa,
this tropical inspired dish will transport you to the islands in no time.*

Serves 4

. . . .

COCONUT CAULIFLOWER RICE

1 medium head of cauliflower

1 cup finely shredded coconut

3 tablespoons cold-pressed coconut oil

1/4 cup chopped cilantro leaves

juice of 1/2 lime

1 large clove of garlic, minced

3/4 teaspoon Himalayan salt

Roughly chop the cauliflower. Place half of it in the food processor and pulse to chop into rice-sized grains. Do not overprocess. Scrape into a large bowl and repeat with the remaining cauliflower. Scrape the rest of the cauliflower into the bowl. Add the coconut, coconut oil, cilantro, lime juice, garlic, and salt to the bowl and mix very well.

MANGO SALSA

1 1/2 cups chopped ripe mango

1 cup diced red bell pepper

1/4 cup diced red onion

1/4 cup chopped cilantro leaves

juice of 1/2 lime

1/2 teaspoon chili powder

1/8 teaspoon salt

Toss all ingredients in a medium bowl and mix well to combine the flavors.

To serve: Divide the rice and salsa into four equal portions. Place the rice on each plate followed by a hearty serving of mango salsa.

TOMATO TOWERS
WITH BRAZIL-BASIL CHEESE
AND MARINATED ARUGULA

*This is a gorgeous dish, smothering thick tomato slices
with a rich, herby Brazil nut cheese and topping them
off with fresh marinated arugula.
This is sure to impress!*

Serves 4–6

- -

BRAZIL-BASIL CHEESE

4 cups water

2¹/2 cups raw Brazil nuts

¹/4 cup cold-pressed olive oil

2 cloves of garlic, minced

1 tablespoon fresh lemon juice

³/4 teaspoon Himalayan salt

¹/2 teaspoon miso

¹/3 cup chopped basil leaves

Place the water and Brazil nuts in a high-speed blender and blend well. Using a nut milk bag or several layers of cheesecloth, strain the nut pulp to remove all of the liquid. Place the remaining Brazil nut milk in the refrigerator to use for smoothies or to replace traditional dairy milk in another recipe.

Take the remaining Brazil nut pulp and place it in your food processor. Add the olive oil, garlic, lemon, salt and miso. Process until all ingredients are well combined. Lastly, add the basil and pulse to combine.

MARINATED ARUGULA

6 cups baby arugula leaves

1/4 cup cold-pressed olive oil

juice of 1/2 lemon

2 cloves of garlic, minced

1/4 teaspoon Himalayan salt

Toss all ingredients in a large bowl and set aside to marinate.

To serve: 4 large tomatoes, cut into 1/2" thick rounds

For each Tomato Tower, place a tomato slice on a plate and top with a generous scoop of Brazil-Basil Cheese. Top with an additional tomato slice and another scoop of cheese. Top it all off with the marinated arugula and serve.

● ● ●

KALE PARCELS WITH DILLY CAULIFLOWER RICE

Using big green leaves to wrap and roll is a living food staple. This fresh dish hides a Mediterranean inspired cauliflower "rice" inside of marinated kale leaves for a unique and satisfying main dish.

Serves 4

KALE PARCELS

1/4 cup cold-pressed olive oil

2 tablespoons fresh lemon juice

1/4 teaspoon Himalayan salt

1 bunch Lacinato kale

In a large bowl, whisk together the olive oil, lemon, and salt. Wash, dry and trim the stems from the kale. Toss the kale leaves in the dressing and set aside to marinate.

DILLY CAULIFLOWER RICE

2¹/₂ cups roughly chopped cauliflower

2¹/₂ cups roughly chopped carrots

¹/₄ cup diced sweet onion

¹/₄ cup chopped dill

¹/₄ cup finely chopped sundried tomatoes
(soak for 4 hours and
drain before chopping)

¹/₄ teaspoon allspice

¹/₄ teaspoon black pepper

1 cup raw macadamia nuts

¹/₂ cup cold-pressed olive oil

2 tablespoons fresh lemon juice

2 cloves garlic

¹/₂ teaspoon Himalayan salt

Place the cauliflower in the food processor and pulse to chop into rice sized grains. Do not overprocess. Repeat with the carrots. Place the cauliflower and carrots in a large bowl and toss with the onion, dill, sundried tomatoes, allspice, and black pepper. Place the macadamia nuts, olive oil, lemon juice, garlic, and salt in the food processor and process to make a paste. Scrape into the cauliflower mixture and mix very well.

To serve: Lay your marinated kale leaves on a cutting board. Divide the Dilly Cauliflower Rice equally among the kale leaves. Roll up the leaves with the rice inside and place on plates to serve.

FETTUCCINE & SHITAKE ALFREDO

Pasta made from ribbons of zucchini is a living food favorite.
It's all about the sauce here with a rich pine nut cream
and meaty marinated mushrooms.

Serves 2–4

. . . .

ZUCCHINI PASTA

6 large zucchini, peeled

1/4 teaspoon Himalayan salt

Using a vegetable peeler, create long strips of zucchini fettuccine about one-quarter to a half-inch wide. Keep rotating the zucchini so that you are peeling all edges rather than continuously peeling in the same spot. When you get to the center of the zucchini and it becomes quite seedy, stop peeling and set aside for use in another recipe. Place the zucchini noodles in a colander and sprinkle with the salt. Toss well and let sit to drain some of the water.

SHITAKE ALFREDO SAUCE

1 1/2 cups shitake mushrooms

1/3 cup coconut aminos, Nama Shoyu,
or wheat-free tamari

1/2 cup pure water

2 cloves of garlic

1/4 cup fresh lemon juice

3/4 teaspoon Himalayan salt

1 1/4 cup raw pine nuts or cashews

Freshly ground black pepper, to serve

Clean and thinly slice the mushrooms. Place in a medium bowl and cover with coconut aminos. Let the mushrooms marinate while you prepare the rest of the sauce. Place the water, garlic, lemon, salt, and nuts in a high-speed blender and blend until very creamy. Pour into a large bowl. Drain the mushrooms (they should now be quite soft) and add to the sauce.

To serve: Press the zucchini noodles to release any last bit of liquid. Add the noodles to the sauce and toss well. Top generously with fresh ground black pepper when serving.

• ● •

LIVE CABBAGE TACOS WITH AVOCADO SALSA

Crunchy, spicy, and super fresh—what more could you ask for in a taco?

Serves 4

• •

TACO SHELLS

8 cabbage leaves

TACO CRUMBLE

1/4 cup coconut aminos, Nama Shoyu, or wheat-free tamari

1/4 cup diced onion

3 cups of raw Sunflower Seeds

4 teaspoons cumin

2 teaspoons ground coriander

1 teaspoon oregano

1/4 teaspoon ground chipotle chili

1/4 cup cilantro leaves, chopped

Place the onion and coconut aminos in a small bowl to marinate. Process the sunflower seeds in a food processor until crumbly. Place the sunflower seeds in a larger bowl and toss with spices and cilantro. Pour the marinated onion over the seed mixture and toss well to combine.

AVOCADO SALSA

2 large tomatoes, diced

1 ripe avocado, diced

1/4 cup chopped cilantro

2 tablespoons diced onion

2 cloves of garlic, minced

2 teaspoons lime juice

1/4 – 1/2 teaspoon Himalayan salt

Mix all ingredients in a medium-sized bowl. Taste for seasoning and adjust if necessary.

To assemble: Divide the Taco Crumble evenly between all of the cabbage leaves. Top each taco off with a generous serving of Avocado Salsa.

● ● ●

SPRING ROLLS WITH SPICY CASHEW DIPPING SAUCE

These fresh and crunchy green rolls are brought to another level with their sweet and spicy cashew dipping sauce.

Serves 4

Spring Rolls

8 large collard leaves, stems removed
and cut in half the long way

5 cups shredded cabbage

2 cups shredded carrot

2 red bell peppers, cut into thin strips

1 container of sprouts, any variety

1/2 cup fresh mint leaves

2 ripe avocados, cut into thin strips

1/4 cup sesame seeds

Place the collard leaves on a cutting board. Divide all the filling ingredients equally, topping the leaves with cabbage, carrots, bell pepper, sprouts, mint, and avocado. Sprinkle with sesame seeds. Roll each wrap neatly and set aside.

Spicy Cashew Dipping Sauce

2 cups raw cashews

1/2 cup cold-pressed sesame oil

1/4 cup water

1/4 cup coconut aminos, Nama Shoyu
or wheat-free tamari

3 cloves of garlic

1 1/4 teaspoon grated ginger

2 tablespoons raw honey

1/2 teaspoon crushed chili pepper

Place all ingredients in a food processor and process until smooth. Serve on the side of the rolls for dipping.

DIVINE DESSERTS

CASHEW CACAO CLUSTERS

*When you need dessert in a hurry, these decadent bites
are your answer. A little crunch and a lot of chocolaty
sweetness make these treats irresistible.*

Makes 16 pieces

. . . .

1/4 cup raw coconut oil (melted)

1/4 cup raw agave nectar

1/3 cup raw cacao powder

pinch of Himalayan salt

3/4 cup raw cashews

2/3 cup coconut flakes

1/4 cup goji berries or raisins

In a medium bowl, whisk together the coconut oil, agave, cacao, and salt. When the chocolate is smooth, add the cashews, coconut, and goji berries or raisins to the bowl. Mix well to coat all of the nuts, coconut, and dried fruit. Use a spoon to create clusters about 2" in diameter and place onto a wax paper lined baking sheet. Freeze 30 minutes or until the chocolate has hardened. Store frozen.

CHOCOLATE MINT TRUFFLES

*These are the perfect size for when you just need a small,
sweet bite. Store them in the freezer so you always have
something to satisfy your chocolate cravings.*

Makes 2 dozen

• •

2 cups raw walnuts

3/4 cup raw cacao powder

pinch of Himalayan salt

1/4 teaspoon organic peppermint extract

15 soft medjool dates, pitted

2 tablespoons raw honey

additional raw cacao powder for coating

Place the walnuts, cacao powder, and salt in the food processor and process until finely ground. Add the peppermint extract, dates, and honey and process again until a smooth dough is formed. Sprinkle some additional cacao powder on a plate. Roll the dough into 1-inch round truffles. Roll each truffle in the cacao powder and place on a dish. Continue until you have used all of the dough. Place in the freezer for 30 minutes to set. Thaw 10 minutes before serving. Store frozen.

• • •

CHERRY CHOCOLATE CHEESECAKE

*Raw, cashew-based cheesecakes are so special, you shouldn't
wait another day before you indulge! Here a creamy
vanilla base is swirled with sweet cherries and is perfectly
complemented by a chocolate crust. Welcome to dessert heaven!*

Makes one 9-inch round cheesecake

. . . .

CRUST

1 cup raw Brazil nuts

1/4 cup cacao

3 tablespoons agave nectar

1 tablespoon coconut oil

pinch salt

Pulse the Brazil nuts in your food processor until finely ground. Add remaining ingredients and process until a sticky dough forms. Press into the bottom of a 9-inch round spring form pan. Place in the freezer to set.

FILLING

3 cups of raw cashews,
soaked for 2 hours in pure water,
drained and rinsed

3/4 cup water

1/4 cup fresh lemon juice

3/4 cup raw honey

2 vanilla beans or
1 1/2 teaspoons of vanilla extract

1 cup cold-pressed coconut oil

1 1/2 cups pitted cherries,
cut into quarters

Place all ingredients except for the cherries in a high-speed blender and blend until very smooth. Pour over the chocolate crust. Add in the cherries and mix to swirl the colors and distribute the cherries. Place in the freezer for 3 hours to set. Once frozen, cut into 8–10 slices and thaw 15 minutes before serving.

Blueberry Coconut Cream Pie

This is a delicious combination of rich coconut cream and sweet blueberries on a lightly spiced almond crust. Simply divine!

Makes one 9-inch pie

. . . .

CRUST

2 cups raw almonds

2 tablespoons raw honey

2 tablespoons raw coconut oil

1/2 teaspoon cinnamon

1/8 teaspoon nutmeg

pinch salt

Process the almonds in a food processor until finely ground. Add all remaining ingredients and process again until well combined.

COCONUT CREAM

2 cups Thai coconut meat

1 vanilla bean or 1/2 teaspoon vanilla extract

1/4 cup raw honey

1/2 cup cold-pressed coconut oil

Place all ingredients in a high-speed bender and blend until very smooth.

SWEET BLUEBERRIES

3 cups blueberries, frozen, thawed, and drained

1/4 cup raw honey

Mix the blueberries and honey in a medium-sized bowl. Let stand for 10 minutes.

To assemble: Press the crust into the bottom and up the sides of a 9-inch pie pan. Cover the crust with one half of the Coconut Cream. Gently strain the blueberries and place them on top of the coconut cream. Top with the remaining Coconut Cream. Refrigerate to set for 4 hours before cutting and serving. Keep frozen for longer storage.

● ● ●

PINA COLADA PIE

This is a beautiful tropical pie, perfect for hot summer days.

Makes one 9-inch pie

· ·

CRUST

1 1/4 cups raw Brazil nuts

3/4 cup coconut flakes

3 tablespoons raw honey

1 tablespoon cold-pressed coconut oil

Place the Brazil nuts and coconut in the food processor and process until finely ground. Add the honey and coconut oil and process again until sticky. Press into the bottom and up the sides of a 9-inch pie pan.

FILLING

1 cup Thai coconut meat

2 cups shredded coconut

1/4 cup raw honey

1/4 cup raw coconut oil

1/2 teaspoon vanilla extract

Place all ingredients in a high-speed blender and blend until smooth. Pour over the crust.

TOPPING

4 cups fresh, ripe pineapple, diced

Pour the pineapple over coconut filling to top the pie. Place in the refrigerator for 4 hours to set before cutting. Freeze for longer storage.

• ● ● •

RASPBERRY CHIA PIE

Sweet, juicy raspberries shine in this bright red pie, held together and made ultra healthy with the magic of chia seeds.

Makes one 9-inch pie

· ·

CRUST

2 cups raw pecans

2 tablespoons raw honey

1 tablespoon cold-pressed coconut oil

1/2 teaspoon cinnamon

pinch salt

Place the pecans in the food processor and process until finely ground. Add all remaining ingredients and process until sticky. Press into the bottom and up the sides of a 9-inch pie pan.

RASPBERRY FILLING

1 cup raspberries (for blending)

1/2 cup raw honey

1 cup raspberries (to be kept whole)

1/2 cup plus 2 tablespoons chia seed

Place 1 cup of raspberries and the honey in the blender and blend until smooth. Pour into a bowl. Fold in the whole raspberries and the chia seed. Pour over the crust and chill 4 hours in the refrigerator to set before serving.

STRAWBERRY TALLCAKE

This layer cake will certainly remind you of strawberry shortcake, though there is nothing short about it! Layers of vanilla cake, coconut vanilla cream, and fresh strawberries stand tall!

Makes one 9-inch cake

CAKE

2¹/₂ cups raw macadamia nuts

1 cup raw cashews

³/₄ cup raw coconut flour

¹/₂ cup raw honey

1 teaspoon vanilla extract

pinch of Himalayan salt

pinch of nutmeg

Process the macadamia nuts and cashews in the food processor until finely ground. Add in the coconut flour, honey, vanilla, salt, and nutmeg, and process again until well combined.

CREAM

2 cups Thai coconut meat

1¹/₂ cups raw cashews,
soaked for 2 hours, drained and rinsed

¹/₂ cup coconut water

¹/₂ cup raw honey

$1/2$ cup raw coconut oil

2 vanilla beans or
$11/2$ teaspoons of vanilla extract

pinch of Himalayan salt

Place all ingredients in a high-speed blender and blend until
very smooth.

STRAWBERRIES

4 cups thinly sliced strawberries

$1/4$ cup raw honey

Mix the strawberries and honey together in a large bowl.

To assemble: Divide the cake, cream and strawberries in half.
Press half of the cake into the bottom of a 9-inch springform
pan. Top with half of the cream followed by half of the strawberries. Repeat with the remaining ingredients until you have
six layers. Refrigerate for 4 hours to set before cutting. Place
in the freezer for longer storage.

CONCLUSION

So here we are. I truly hope you are excited about the prospect of utilizing Slender GR™ to help you lose weight. The fact that it is a 100-percent natural substance with no specter of negative side effects looming over it surely has to put your mind at ease and increase your positive expectations.

Naturally, it is my sincerest desire that what you have read here about the dietary possibilities I presented in support of Slender GR™ has resonated with you—at least to the degree that you will give them a try. I say this because as much as I would like to see you reach your goals in terms of the weight you wish to shed, it is equally important to me that you experience an overall improvement in your health. The good news is it's all connected; the body works on *all* levels simultaneously. Whether it's excess weight, sleep issues, digestive problems, skin troubles, general aches and pains, or serious illness, the body doesn't discriminate and work on one issue and not another, or only work on one issue depending upon existing circumstances. The nature of the living body is to work on everything equally all the time. So if you are eating intelligently, you are supplying the body with what it needs to work, thereby strengthening and supporting the body's effort in total.

I know how daunting a challenge it can be sometimes listening to a legion of people deemed to be authorities, including me, who all have differing opinions about a subject for which no one has all the answers. It is for that very reason that I went to such great lengths to instill in you what may be a newfound reverence and appreciation for the incomparable intelligence that governs your body and all that it does. Above all else, your living body strives to operate at optimum efficiency and to experience long-term, uninterrupted, pain-free, good health. And if we can simply learn how to effectively get out of the way and support, rather than interfere with, those efforts, good health is precisely what will occur. We were not put here and given the gift of life only to suffer every possible malady imaginable. That is abnormal and unnatural. The *natural* inclination of the living body is a lasting and unwavering state of well-being.

Why is it, then, that so few people are enjoying such an exalted state of health? So many people are overweight and unwell. It has even begun to affect children in unprecedented numbers. More children are overweight than ever before. An ever-increasing number of children are dealing with chronic health conditions like diabetes and asthma. Developmental disabilities such as autism, ADD (attention deficit disorder), and ADHD (attention deficit hyperactivity disorder) are skyrocketing. Why? I'll tell you why I think it is happening, and it won't be a surprise to you from what you have read here—it's due to our progressively deteriorating diets.

It is for this reason why it is so essential that adults learn how to eat healthfully and support healthy digestion—*so it can be passed on to children.* I just mentioned autism, a subject with which I have become increasingly interested. According to every available statistical resource, autism is the fastest-growing developmental disorder in the United States, with a new diagnosis every fifteen to twenty minutes! One of the people leading the way in helping some of our most challenged members of society is Dr. Phillip DeMio, executive director of the American Medical Autism Board. Dr. DeMio has been using and researching the use of digestive enzymes in children dealing with autism in his clinics for the past number of years, with outstanding results.

Here is what Dr. DeMio has to say on this subject: "Virtually each and every person on the Autism Spectrum has digestive problems. In the ASD (autism spectrum disorder) community, the need for nutritional direction and gut support is imperative. *Some 80% of children and adults on the spectrum report severe digestive issues.* The goal of every parent is to give their children the highest quality of life. By making some important dietary changes and adding digestive enzymes, our findings are that many of our children and adults are greatly aided and improve their digestion. This alleviated distress can then lead to a number of other improvements. The goal remains to get the word out; there *is* hope and relief for these youngsters and adults that are suffering. I feel strongly that by assisting the digestive difficulties many are dealing with, we can help families achieve a better quality of life for our kids."

These days there seems to be a plot afoot, be it intentional or accidental, to keep us ill fed, poorly nourished, and ever more dependent upon a vast array of pharmaceuticals in order to combat the inevitable result of prolonged, inferior nutrition. People are routinely convinced to eat foods promoted by slick advertising campaigns that label them as natural, wholesome, and nutritious—when they are no more natural, wholesome, and nutritious than a barrel of MSG! The nutritive quality of our food is increasingly substandard. It's highly processed and no longer resembles anything that ever grew naturally out of the ground. And that shortchanges us on the very nutrition we rely upon that food to provide.

I think because we are under such an assault all the time from marketers and public relations, experts to "eat this," "do that," "listen to your doctor," and "take this medicine," that we somehow have become disconnected from, and lost faith in, the inherent dynamics of the living body. There is a huge, fundamental difference between the standard medical approach (allopathy) and that of natural healing (orthopathy). Mainstream medicine looks at the human body as a hapless, helpless victim, forever at the mercy of any and all malevolent forces that may attack it and lay it low. Not so with the natural approach, which is largely ignored or dismissed, and which views the living body as dynamic, as being *fully* capable of caring for itself and maintaining itself when honored and supported to do so.

In terms of diagnosis and treatment, the medical standard is run like a gristmill. Generally speaking, doctors record your symptoms, look up the typical treatment, prescribe the appropriate drug, and send you on your way—next! I can tell you, after studying this stuff for more than forty years, that the biggest mistake in people's thinking, and the biggest hurdle to overcome, is the idea that when something uncomfortable is going on with the body it is something bad happening *to* the body rather than something *good* the body initiated and is doing for itself. As regards the living body and its well-being, there is no greater lesson to learn.

I will readily acknowledge that it is a difficult concept to accept for people who have been conditioned all their lives to believe otherwise, but in actual fact almost all so-called diseases have a similar cause, differentiated only by where in the body they occur. That cause is the accumulation of uneliminated wastes (toxins). What is most encouraging and liberating is the fact that—and once again, despite efforts to convince you otherwise—the remedy for all of these alleged ailments comes down to supporting the living body in its ongoing efforts to cleanse and heal itself of anything not supportive of overall health.

Thankfully, that is what the body is *always* doing. Always! It is something the living body does for its own survival twenty-four hours a day. Food doesn't heal, pills and potions don't heal, special ingredients in certain herbs don't heal, supplements don't heal, and drugs don't heal. Healing of the body takes place *by* the body when it is provided with the care and treatment it needs to strengthen and support all of its activities, and it is our obligation to get out of the body's way and not impede its efforts.

The means by which each of us can accomplish the lofty goal of good health, which includes reaching and maintaining a healthy weight, is not nearly as complicated as many people have been led to believe. All it requires is the utilization of a few basic, well-proven, and time-tested principles—mainly a decidedly nutritious diet consisting of a sensible amount of living, uncooked food, support of the body's cleansing and healing mechanism (the lymph system), regular exercise, and avoidance of drugs. So much talk, conjecture, and complexity have been piled on top of these few, simple, straightforward principles that people have been made to feel overwhelmed, if not helpless, in acquiring what has been misconstrued as being nearly beyond their reach—lifelong good health and well-being.

If I were to say to you that, "in addition to having antecubital and retropopliteal urticaria with pruritis, a sphygmomanometer indicates orthostatic hypertension," would you know what I meant? It means that in addition to itchy arms and legs a blood pressure test indicates dizziness. Why not just say that instead of the alphabet soup?

No one had to read this book with a dictionary and a physiology textbook by his or her side merely to understand what was being said. I have intentionally kept it nontechnical and easy to read so that you can feel more at ease and less exasperated with a subject all too often presented in a fashion that prevents the message from being clearly understood. It's so important that you come to realize that the living body is enormously responsive to improved treatment, ever ready to do whatever needs doing in order to both acquire and maintain a consistent level of health and well-being for itself.

These efforts of the body to which I am referring do *not* need to be forced into activity but rather simply unleashed. If you are in a state of ill health, the body will persistently marshal its forces in a tireless quest to restore health. And once achieved, the body automatically directs those very same forces and efforts toward maintaining that state. That's how the body works. It can do nothing else.

Have you ever seen a horse race like the Kentucky Derby? Before the starting gates are opened, those 1,000-pound animals are stomping, snorting, and bucking in eager anticipation of being let loose. The very *instant* the gate is removed from their path all they want to do is blast around that race track as fast as their legs and lungs will allow with every ounce of strength and heart they possess. They don't casually trot around the track as though they were out for a laid-back walk; it is an all-or-nothing, full on gallop to that finish line as though their lives were at stake.

That effort of the horse can be likened to your body's nonstop quest to achieve health in the quickest, most efficient way possible. That's all it knows how to do, and the only way to keep it from its appointed task is by depriving it of the living food it needs or by overwhelming it with more toxins than it can eliminate—or doing both. And *even then* the body will never give up its efforts; so long as it is alive, the body is on a one-pointed pursuit of well-being. It is the choices you make that will determine its failure or success. So eager is your body to do the best for itself that even a moderate improvement will reap noticeable rewards.

To the very best of my ability I have imparted herein what you can do to increase the likelihood of keeping your weight in check, feeling good, having a lot of energy, remaining well, and not becoming a medical statistic. And it's not as though the recommendations I am suggesting will throw your life into turmoil or cause you to feel deprived. On the contrary, they are exceedingly easy and simple to incorporate into your lifestyle and are very forgiving. Plus—they prove their worth and effectiveness in short order.

Obviously, Slender GR™ does a good amount of the work for you in terms of losing excess weight. But beyond that, what I am saying is that by simply increasing the amount of living food you eat, eating fruit until noon, and separating proteins from starches as often as is convenient, along with some moderate exercise, you can revolutionize your life. You can fully enjoy the eating experience without "dieting" and still look and feel wonderful. I am asking you to just *try*, for a while, doing what I suggest to see if what I am saying is true.

Remember what I said earlier—*millions* of people have taken me up on my challenge and have benefited from doing so. They are using the principles I shared to the degree they desire and in a way convenient for their particular lifestyle—and they are flourishing. There is no reason on earth why you cannot join their ranks. This is what I wish for you with all my heart.

Afterword

A Note from
Toby Coriell

Toby Coriell is currently the President of V.P. Consultants Inc. (www.vpnutrition.com), a company specializing in providing both education and products associated with preventive care and natural supplementation. He has conducted seminars and consulted at the corporate level both nationally and internationally. Mr. Coriell has been closely associated with Harvey Diamond and Fit For Life over the past fifteen years. His interests in supplementation and preventative care have been a driving force behind his actively consulting with leaders in the Natural Foods industry. He has consulted and partnered with FEMA in providing food, water, and shelter for victims of natural disasters throughout the United States. Currently he is the Managing Director of the Autism Hope Alliance (AHA). AHA is a nonprofit organization that sprung forth from the Natural Foods Industry. Its goal is to educate the public in finding appropriate nutrition and care for families dealing with Autism Spectrum Disorder and assisting with the care of children.

It does not happen often in life that you come across an individual who has the personal determination to stay true to his core beliefs and yet is open to new and different ideas. Someone who sticks to their convictions and marches through life's ups and downs with the same optimistic mind-set as if it were just another good day to be alive. Such has been my personal experience over the past couple of decades with Harvey Diamond.

When I first met Harvey I was attending one of his seminars, listening to him speak about good health practices. As I watched and listened, I thought, *He is not being presented in a manner that his message deserves.*

I made that comment to someone involved in putting the evening together, thought nothing more of it, and left. A few days later, I received a call from Harvey inviting me over to speak with him at his home. Someone had given him my business card. After speaking for a bit, Harvey asked if I would be interested in working with him in the publishing of his next book. Thus started our journey as friends and business associates, one that has lasted over many years.

Through the years of our being associated, raising families, going through illness, economic problems, and everything else we all deal with, Harvey has maintained his positive outlook on life. Not just his own life, but also those lives he has touched through his writing. I have worked with him on numerous book releases, television appearances, and radio shows. Even when it seemed like there was no real "business" advantage to being involved in a project, through it all, Harvey has always been focused on conveying his message wherever and whenever he can: "You have the right to better health."

In reviewing letters and emails from around the globe, many where it is evident that there is no real "commercial advantage" to answering it, Harvey will spend the same amount of time with each individual. Just like his books, he takes a very personal interest in those who seek him out for advice. That one aspect of his personality has led me to conclude that he really just wants to help people, and as you will read here, he has been a success at that for years.

This is not designed as the "Harvey for President" part of the book. Sometimes, the adulation of others has an alternative motive involved. I assure you that is not the case here. When I was asked to contribute my thoughts to the latest literary work for Harvey, I was honored. Not for any other reason than this: With all of the apathetic, self-serving people on this planet, I felt like taking the opportunity to tell a little about the better side of humanity; one of the people dedicated to helping others. When was the last time you sat down to watch the evening news and it was full of nothing but positive, uplifting news? Or when did you see a story on constructive personal profiles that make a difference in other people's lives. They are out there, but sadly, far and few between. Harvey's story may not make the evening news. However, the millions of people who he has helped all feel differently. I am happy to share a number of their short messages with you in the following few pages.

As mentioned, these unsolicited comments from people do not tell the whole story. Imagine someone that you have never met and who does not know you or your family. That person takes time to help you and maybe even steer you in a direction that you feel saves your life or the life of one of your loved ones. That is an impact that is incalculable in value. Harvey has been that same person over the years, and has the letters and thank-you notes to prove it. Now, in our "what is newsworthy" society, that may not sound like a story. But if you ask me, we need more stories like that. Who knows, maybe this will make the evening news? I hope so.

· · · · ·

Dear Harvey,

This is not an inquiry, but rather a thank you. I read *Fit For Life* twenty years ago and it changed my life overnight. I made my first smoothie (one of thousands since), went outside, and sat in the sun (for the first time without feeling afraid), and I was hooked. It would take a long time to tell you the impact your book has had on my life, and through me, on the lives of my children and my extended family. I just felt like I needed to thank you. I'm forever grateful to you and the work that you do.

Sincerely,

J.S.

Dear Harvey,

I just wanted to tell you my *Fit For Life* story. I found your book (*Fit For Life*) at my parents' house in 1990. I read it in two days and I started correctly combining my foods and found that the less meat I ate the better I felt. I soon stopped eating meat. Two years later I met my wife, and she was always getting sick. She started eating the *Fit For Life* way and started feeling so good that she has been eating this way for the eighteen years we have been together. We have two children that we are raising this way as well. I am a chef and was not eating very well at work and found myself not feeling very well and had a growing waistline. I changed jobs and my new restaurant had a juice bar (Foodlife in Chicago), and I broke out all your books and started juicing. Then I heard about "p90x" on the radio and started eating the Fit For Life way and working out. I lost 4 inches off my waist (now a size 30), and 40 pounds, going from 26 percent body fat to 13 percent. I am 44 years old and run circles around people half my age. I just wanted to say thank you for once again changing my life for the better and making a difference in my family's health and future well-being.

—L.D.

* * * * *

Dear Harvey,

I want to thank you for your book *Fit For Life*. I just started the program—ten days ago—and have lost 3 pounds. I am very interested in the food combining the most. I have also said good-bye to dairy, flour, and sugar. I cannot tell you how much better I feel already. I was to the point that when I awakened in the morning my first thought was, "I can't wait to get back home tonight and go to bed." Exhaustion, stomach issues, feelings of defeat . . . Now I am up, ready to greet the day, and feel energized throughout the day. And I now sleep better than ever.

Thank You. Thank You. Grace and Peace

—G.F.

Dear Mr. Diamond,

I would like to thank you, Harvey Diamond, for the impact you've had on my life and way of thinking. The first time I read *Fit For Life*, I was only nine years old (I'm now twenty-five). Inspired by my older brothers' example, and my athletic lifestyle, you made me aware and curious about the effect and impact of nutrition on my body and lifestyle. I have not always followed the guidelines of natural hygiene—sometimes not at all. However, I feel the greatest gift you've given is the knowledge and the permission not to be perfect. Also, you have made me understand the importance of being healthy and not just having a great figure.

Nowadays, I strive to give my body the fuel it needs. The number-one guideline that I follow is the principle of eating fruit correctly. I love the feeling of fruit in an empty stomach; I can almost feel how beautifully it works inside me.

Thank you again, and I wish all the best for you!

Hugs,

—R.J.

. . . . .

Dear Mr. Diamond,

Just a quick note to add my voice to the many, many others who have given you well-deserved praise. I have never read a book on health-related issues as though it were an engrossing novel that I couldn't put down. Over the years I've had many pieces of the puzzle, but until I read *Fit For Life: A New Beginning*, I wasn't able to put them all together. You have enabled me to do so and for that I am eternally grateful. I found it especially gratifying to hear the spiritual aspect of your endeavors; you are truly a complete human being. I wish you continued success and from the bottom of my heart, I thank you.

—J.J.

. . . . .

Hi Harvey,

I immensely appreciate your kind and generous heart in answering my letter! No wonder people say amazing things about you. Only a heart that has been exposed somehow to God's compassion and mercy can reply the way you did.

I have been promoting and spreading the message of your books among the people at my church, and many other churches also invite me to do so. I have talked about your work with confidence, and your book has been advertised faithfully in most of my conferences with few exceptions. I hope to see more books coming out of your pen on that line.

Be blessed,

—M.B.

• • • • •

Dear Mr. Diamond,

When your book first came out, I was in high school and had stomachaches all the time. I was raised on an organic farm and we had quality food, air, and water. Later, I married and started a family. I am now forty-two and have tried everything to lose the weight that I gained from having my two children.

Several weeks ago, my neighbor had a garage sale and was selling *Fit For Life*. I got it thinking, "Why not give it a shot?" I can't believe the difference it has made in my life! No stomachaches! I'm losing weight! I'm not miserable! And, had I known all the info in that book plus in *Fit For Life II* (which I bought new.), I would have raised my kids differently and known a little more about the medical system, food industry, and so forth.

I have recommended your book to all my friends. My husband and mother also follow your plan. We just tweaked it to fit our schedules, cooking styles, and so on. It is so EASY!

Had someone told me that I'd get to the point where I didn't really care about "splurge" meals, I would have laughed at them! My husband and I joke that the worse trouble we can get into at "our age" is ill-combining a meal!

Thanks so much; you are still reaching people.

—C.M.

Dear Harvey,

In the 1980s when *Fit For Life* arrived on the shelves, I excitedly purchased the book and followed the program. I lost a lot of weight and inches and felt amazing. But, like anyone who is young, I wasn't able to stick with it and regained my weight. Over the years I tried way too many diets. I lost and gained a ton of weight and my body was taking a beating from all these diets that did not teach me anything but how to yo-yo diet.From childhood I suffered with irritable bowel syndrome.In 1987, after an ectopic pregnancy and surgery, my stomach problems worsened. I suffered chronic digestive problems and was unable to digest food for way too many years. I tried so many things for the pain, and lived my life around my sensitive stomach. Five years ago I ended up with food poisoning, and the problems with my digestion worsened, increasing my weight gain. I was on a lot of medication, which worsened my already sensitive stomach problems.

In April 2010, a friend lost a lot of weight incorporating food-combining principals. She told me of your program, which she was following. A lightbulb went on and immediately I dug out my *Fit For Life* book. I knew it worked before, and I was truly ready this time to alter my life for the long haul. I was tired of suffering constant weight gain, gluten sensitivity, dairy allergy, and the endless weight rollercoaster. Simply put, I was tired of dieting!

That day changed my life. It was so easy to return to *Fit For Life,* the weight was dropping, and I started to digest my food. It was a miracle. I am down 20 pounds since April and feel wonderful. Harvey, you absolutely found the key to curing obesity, as well as digestive disorders. The difference in my overall body is a miracle. My husband has lost three pants sizes and likes this way of eating because he does not sense deprivation.

I am forever grateful to you Harvey for this life-saving *Fit For Life* program. I eat fruit until noon and food combine throughout my day. I have more energy and have not taken any antacids or stomach medicine since I started back on this lifesaving program. Thank you, Harvey, for this program that has saved my life.

Sincerely and with thanks,

—B.L.

Hi!

I have been on "fit for life" for about four days and I feel so much better and have a lot of energy. It really works. Everybody should be on "fit for life." It really makes sense.

Thank you very much,

—H.R.

· · · · ·

Dear Harvey,

I'm pretty sure you have saved my life! I was diagnosed with RA one year ago, but I have reason to believe there were much darker forces working in my body (possibly rectal or colon with the pain I was having). When I received the phone call that I had RA, I immediately started a two-week juice fast (thanks to the information I read in one of your books). I have been eating only living food for the past year and juicing for seven days every three weeks.

I had planned to do this for six months, but when that time came and the pain was still there I decided to go for a year.

Well, tomorrow will be a year and all the pain is virtually gone.

Just saying "thank you" doesn't seem enough for what you've done for me.

God bless you,

—D.M.

· · · · ·

Hello Harvey,

I just picked up your book four days ago. I started on a new lifestyle plan thirty days back, and I am so excited to read and understand what you have said in your book *Fit For Life* (1985 edition).

I am a single mom of a four-year-old boy, and I have let myself slide. In the last thirty days I lost 5.6 kg, but I feel so motivated now that I have read your book. I know that this will be a change for the better.

Thank you for all you have done. I am so excited as I start this journey of losing weight and gaining well-being. I had hoped to

reach my goal weight of 65 kg by June, but I bet with the FFL program it will be way sooner!!
Thank you!
—C.

· · · · ·

Hello, Mr. Diamond,

I'm just writing to say thank you about twenty years too late. A waiter at the restaurant where I was a busboy recommended *Fit For Life* to me when I was just eighteen years old. All these years (and many life changes, including a difficult divorce) later, I am still very often reminded of particular turns of phrase and images you created in the original book that literally changed my life for the better. I became a writer and teacher (not related to health, but am starting a new blog next month) with many thanks to you and your transformational research and writing in the 1970s and 1980s. I trust you and your family are well; and thank you again.
—T. E.

· · · · ·

Hi Mr. Diamond

I have recently read your book and absolutely loved it! It made so much sense. I have been trying as much as possible to follow the correct eating behavior within the time brackets. Thank you for the great health tips—certainly a life-changing book!
—L.

· · · · ·

Dear Harvey,

I have had your books for many years. I am re-reading *Fit For Life* and *Fit For Life II*.

Gosh, they are awesome. Bringing all the information together under one cover. It makes sense. I followed your method for many years and then, through a series of unfortunate events, fell away and fell ill. Now, back on track, and although I still have a long way to go,

I'm combining and ingesting fresh and sometimes even organic f's and v's.

What a difference! OMG, not to feel bloated and miserable, joint pain gone completely, and on and on. I end up eating more pound for pound of veggies and fruit than of meats and dairy and feel so light and fit and filled with energy (same as before . . . duhhh)

Thanks so very much for your studies and for bringing it all together for us.

—B.

. . . . .

Hello Harvey,

I recently discovered your *Fit For Life* book and have been amazed and educated by the many insights and information on natural hygiene and so forth. The information is even more relevant today than ever! I really can't put it into words how engaged I am in the material. Thank you for doing this so many years ago. It is a great contribution to people, especially in America. I hope you are well and just wanted you to know your book is still making a difference.

Only wish I had found it years ago.

Best regards,

—S. K.

. . . . .

To Fit For Life,

I don't really have an enquiry, I just wanted to let Harvey know that I have your original *Fit For Life* book, which I bought in 1985, and I have adopted most of the principles with success. I am now forty-nine years old and for the last couple of years am experiencing menopausal symptoms plus extra unwanted pounds that keep creeping up. I have tried protein diets and other diets with no results, but I have to admit I pulled out my old faithful *Fit For Life* book and am reading it again. So I just wanted to let you know that your theory— much to some skeptic's surprise—DOES WORK!

—R. K.

. . . . .

Dear Harvey,

Years ago I found your book in a book club offer. I bought *Fit For Life* and read it cover to cover in hours. I was curious about how sure you were that it worked. In the book you challenge everyone to try it for two weeks and if we feel better on our old eating habits, go back to them. I thought okay, I can do two weeks. I did everything you said to a T. I was hooked. In one month I lost 23 pounds and my health improved. My skin glowed and my energy was out of this world. I just bought a new copy (again) of your book, and I am starting out again with it knowing how much better I will feel. I have three beautiful daughters and slipped into the old habits I grew up with—fast, processed food—and boy have I paid for it. You saved my life and made it wonderful once, and I know it is going to happen again, and my daughters will benefit also. Thank you from the bottom of my heart for your caring and the love that you put into your research. You have improved many people's lives through me. I bet I have given 100 or more of your books as gifts over the years and told twice as many people about it.

I just wanted to say thanks again.

—K .M

• • • • •

Hello Mr. Diamond,

Thanks for all you share in your quest for good health for humanity. I am currently reading your book, *Fit For Life,* and have found it a wonderful confirmation of many things shared over the years.

—L. A.

• • • • •

I would like to thank you, Harvey, for your *Fit For Life* books. I have them all and to be honest they are the only books that make sense to me. Every chapter is so well explained.

Thank you.

—L. F.

• • • • •

Dear Mr. Diamond,

For almost twenty years now I have been a keen follower of recommendations enclosed in the *Fit For Life* books. I think it's natural,
simple, and just brilliant.
—A. J.

•　•　•　•　•

Dear Mr. Diamond,

I have read your book *Fit For Life, Not Fat For Life* and I thought
it wonderful. I adopted the plan and lost 7 lbs and went down one
dress size.
—S. R.

•　•　•　•　•

Dear Harvey,

I recently bought your book *Fit For Life* from Amazon, after so
many great recommendations from friends, and I must say it lived up
to the reputation. Great book! Now I want to share this treasure and
all the tips included in the book with my family, who I believe can
really benefit from what you are preaching.
—P. C.

•　•　•　•　•

Dear Harvey,

I own and have read all your books and am a strong believer in
fruit until noon. I have been doing that premise along with eating
mostly living foods and have seen amazing health improvements:
reversing diabetes and chronic fatigue and lowering blood pressure to
normal. I am off all meds.
—M. L.

•　•　•　•　•

Dear Mr. Diamond,

I was introduced to the *Fit For Life* lifestyle about ten years ago,
and my life has been truly enriched and enhanced by this knowledge.
Thank you for your commitment to truly helping people with their
overall health and well-being!
—L. F.

I would like to thank Harvey Diamond and his book *Fit For Life*. I followed the eating habits outlined in the book, not to the letter, but close enough to lose seventy-five pounds in a year and two months.
—R. C.

*   *   *   *   *

Dear Harvey—

Your books, *Fit For Life, Not Fat For Life* and *Fit For Life: A New Beginning*, are terrific! I have been on the program for one month. I have lost fifteen pounds and never felt better. Energy level is way up and I feel younger and stronger too. It truly is a new beginning. Thank you!
—B. D.

*   *   *   *   *

Hello Mr. Diamond,

I just want to thank you for your books, which really opened my eyes. I immediately started the Mono diet and although it is a big change for me I feel great.

Years ago, I read your first book, *Fit For Life,* and I could not change my lifestyle then. So I was and still am overweight, but now the motivation is different and it really works.

I cannot thank you enough for the great books, and I have bought some more just to give them to friends so they can read them as well.
—N. V. from Finland

*   *   *   *   *

Dear Mr. Diamond,

Keep up the good work. My wife and I have read every one of your books. We have been on your diet for the last fifteen years. Well at least 90 percent. I do still drink coffee, but we eat this tremendous bowl of fruit in the morning.

I have been able to cut my high blood pressure medicine in half. My wife is sixty-seven, I am sixty-eight, and we are able to lead a good, healthy life.

Thanks again for holding the line,
—J. & M.

Hi Harvey,

How are you? I am a Chinese girl from Ningbo, China. Two weeks ago I tried to contact you. The purpose for my call that day is I want to help my fellowmen here to express their gratitude to you. I always read their comment on your book, *Fit For Life*, online. How many times I have read that they want to thank you how for your book *Fit For Life* turned their lives around entirely. As you know, our country is still a developing country. We are still not rich. For most average people, health medical care is unaffordable once they got serious disease. People have to burn their money once they get serious disease. Fortunately, our people found your book at a local bookstore. They believe your concept and employ your health concept in their daily life and their life changed. Some people even organized a juice group to help people know this great way to keep good health condition.

I think I should let you know all this happen in China and let you know how grateful we are to you, the writer of *Fit For Life*. Thank you! By the way, have you ever traveled to China? People who are your reader in China will warmly welcome you to travel here.

So happy,

—P. C.

• • • • •

Dear Harvey,

After being diagnosed with lupus in November 2006, I am so happy to report that I am no longer feeling the crippling effects like I did. I can't say thank you enough for turning me in the right direction to help my body heal. It's truly a miracle, a miracle of the body, and it's a shame more people haven't found this. We all would be so much healthier!!! I am forever grateful to you.

HUGS—my heart to your heart,

—C. L.

• • • • •

Dear Harvey,

I wanted to reach out to you to tell you what a profound impact you have had on me.

Fit For Life not only took away 35 pounds of excess weight and lowered my cholesterol by 85 points, it also opened my eyes to what's going on all around us: overprocessed, genetically altered, HFCS-saturated junk on the shelves in our grocery.

My children will grow up with this same knowledge.

I've been sharing my story and your incredible book with family and many friends. Some have lost as much as 50+ pounds!

Thanks so much for sharing your gift so many years ago. The message is as relevant today as ever.

—G. S.

. . . . .

Hi Harvey:

I have been following *Fit For Life* for two years now. I have eliminated meat from my diet and eat a lot more raw fruit and vegetables (fruit smoothie for breakfast). Because of the change in my diet, I no longer need my medication for underactive thyroid. I wanted to get off my thyroid medication, so my naturopath had me gradually go off my medication, then sent me for some blood work and my thyroid is fine. My eyesight has dramatically improved as well.

Thank you for *Fit For Life*.

—D.C.

. . . . .

Dear Harvey,

Reading *Fit For Life* and following its basic principles has changed my life. Before reading it, I struggled with my weight, all of my life. Not anymore!

I am a fervent believer in your methods and I've been following them for years. Even though I haven't read the book (again) in a very long time, I still remember large portions of it. It made a huge impression on me! Thank you!

Very truly yours,

—E. L.

. . . . .

Dear Harvey,

Not an inquiry, just a huge thank you for your Healthy Weight-Loss plan. I have been on your diet for nearly three months now and have changed the life of my daughter (who I live with) her husband and my grandchild. We love it. Every day we discover something new and there is nothing we don't like. My grandchild, who is now four, has only known cereal and has had no problem in the transition from cereal to fruit. She will come downstairs and say, "I want a banana or mango," or whatever she feels like, but always fruit. I have lost twenty pounds and feel wonderful. I have no desire to put anything into my mouth that does not come from Mother Earth. Thank you ever so much once again for helping us back to our roots (the way God intended).

—J. V.

• • • • •

Dear Harvey,

Over the last ten years I have studied many books on nutrition, and tried many different eating methods.

In reading *Fit For Life, Not Fat For Life*, I feel like I've come to know you on a personal level. It is a delight that in my life I have been given the chance to obtain your knowledge and wisdom around such a simple yet complex subject as food. You are a fair person, and you offer a broad opinion that is backed by common sense and logic. I have been meaning to write to you since first reading *Fit For Life*, and some ten years later I still refer to your books as my manual for life in many cases.

I want you to know that you have made a massive difference to my life and I am sure many others.

You are a great man. Thank you.

—M. A., Adelaide, Australia

• • • • •

Dear Mr. Diamond

I just wanted to say that the day I discovered your book *Fit For Life* was the best day of my life. I always felt there was more to the story of obesity and other health problems than we were being told by so-called experts. But your books have opened my eyes. And I live by your principles every single day. I have concluded that this is the diet that best serves the human body. I was so angry that I had been so misinformed about food and how it affects the body. But your books painted a very clear picture for me. I just want to thank you for what you are doing and encourage you to keep doing it. There are not a lot of people out there who are willing to tell the truth. We need more people like you promoting the true methods of losing weight and being healthy. Thanks again, Mr. Diamond. Keep doing what you do and God bless you.

—C. F.

• • • • •

Dear Harvey,

After running in my eighteenth marathon, I am more fanatical than ever about the *Fit For Life* program. Since I am fifty-nine and a half, almost sixty, I am motivated to the extent that I am personally transcribing, word for word, your original book. Not only do I want the words, but I find that the exercise further instills the information into my being. It will empower me during my weekly run in the morning.

Thanking you,

—M. H.

• • • • •

Dear Mr. Diamond,

I have read every book you have written. I am a "follower" of *Fit For Life*. As I read your original book everything was just clicking. Everything made total and complete sense. The foods we eat, when we eat them, how we eat them, and how we prepare them. I was already a very healthy person as regards to food and exercise, but your books brought it full circle and made everything so much clearer.

So I wanted to thank you and tell you of my good fortune thanks to your books. I am a Weight Watcher leader. I went on Weight Watchers to lose 20 pounds and I did, but it was a pain to keep tracking food and keep the weight off. Since following *Fit For Life* I

have not been tracking the foods I eat, because the foods are living, healthy, and fresh, and I have lost an additional 10 pounds without effort. As you say, SO SIMPLE, so obvious, and so common sense.
Thank you,
—M. H.

·　·　·　·　·

Dear Mr. Diamond,

My husband of thirty years and I received your first book, *Fit For Life,* about ten years ago. We laughed and cried throughout the reading of your book while eating "new" meals of fresh, raw fruits and vegetables. My husband went from 210 to 155 pounds. It wasn't until we received your book *Fit For Life* that we both learned the right way to eat! We are now fifty-one and fifty-three years old and have more energy and stamina than people half our age. Most people think I'm in my thirties, so I just quote my husband and say, "Chronologically I am fifty-one, but biologically I am only thirty-five!"

Mr. Diamond, if more people helped others as much as you have done, this world would be a wonderful, healthy, and happy place to live. Have you ever thought of cloning yourself?
A simple, humble thank you is just not enough to express our appreciation for you. From the bottom of our hearts (and liver and kidneys and appendix), thank you.
—V & R

·　·　·　·　·

Hi Harvey,

I first want to say thanks. WOW, I am almost sad that it took me till I was thirty-seven to find out about this information. FYI: I was 6 feet three inches and 220 pounds, working out semiregularly. The second I heard the tape of your book I began sticking to it with no exceptions whatsoever. Now I am 185 pounds with tons of energy and feel great. I am extremely passionate about this and feel everyone should at least hear something about it.
Thanks,
—J. B.

• • • • •

Dear Mr. Diamond,

I just wanted to let you know that I have been using the *Fit For Life* original book since I was sixteen years old. I am now thirty-seven (in great health by the way). I was introduced to it by a teacher in high school and was amazed at how I felt after the two week program (and I thought I was a healthy individual at the time). It was a rejuvenation—the same as people who who have had long-term pain/illness and it is finally relieved. They (and I) never realized how terrible the pain/sickness was until it was gone.

I had planned to vent my frustration to you of various criticisms I have heard over the years of your method and ideas, but I realized, you have probably heard them all before, and in the end, people will believe what they want regardless of any facts or simple, irrefutable logic you present. So, I will just say to you that I will continue living healthy, thanks to you, and I will continue to promote your theory of healthy, simple living to everyone who is astounded by my age.
Thank you for my life,
—M. C.

• • • • •

Dear Harvey,

I purchased the original *Fit For Life* book probably twenty years ago. I had been on that all-protein diet off and on, trying to lose weight and in the process almost killed myself. I am so excited to be doing this. I have dropped 11 pounds in two weeks and all I do is eat!!! I will keep you posted on my continued success and send before and after pictures some day. Oh, I forgot to mention. I dropped my cholesterol from 178 down to 142 in two weeks. Absolutely amazing! I switched from eggs to fruit in the morning and combining every meal. My doctor is dumbfounded at the fast results and is truly interested in what I am doing. Thank you for such wonderful research and a great plan.
—T. B.

• • • • •

Hi,

I am a male, age 43, and I have applied the ideas Harvey Diamond puts forth in *Fit For Life* and I am in better shape than I have ever been in my life and healthier than I have ever been. I lost over 60 pounds. I used to pop antacids like candy; now, I never use them at all.

Thank you!!

—M. R.

• • • • •

Dear Harvey,

I hope this note reaches you. First, let me say thank you. Thank you for being such an inspiration to me, to my husband, and to our three very healthy and wonderful children. All five of us have read your books, and have been living the very lifestyle you write about, and sharing your wisdom with as many people as possible for many many years. *Fit For Life* changed my husband's and my life seventeen years ago, and we are forever grateful to you.

Thanks for listening, and for your amazing life work.

With admiration and love,

—S. L.

• • • • •

Dear Mr. Diamond,

I'm sure you receive hundreds of emails like this all the time, but here's another one to add to your collection.

I first purchased your book *Fit For Life, Not Fat For Life* at the airport in January of this year (2005). I have tried so many diets over the many years and I thought I would be reading just another diet book. I was pleasantly surprised after reading your book.

Let me tell you, for a woman who was only 98 pounds until I was 30 years old, I thought I could eat anything I wanted. Being 45 years old now and weighing close to 150 pounds, and always yo-yo dieting, I had just about given up on ever being slim again. Since using your method of fruit in the morning and doing about 80 percent raw foods, I have lost 25 pounds and feel and look great. I'm sure I will eventually get the other 10 pounds off that I want. I walk 4 miles a day on the treadmill and have tons of energy now.

This past month I finally kicked my smoking habit that I have had for the last fifteen years. As you wrote in one of your books (I can't remember which one, I have read almost all of them), I just gradually lost the taste for them and decided that was it.

I just wanted to thank you for sharing your knowledge with me. I can't believe how well I feel now. I have had so many people ask me about why I look so good that I share your techniques whenever I can. I even pass out your books, that I have read, to people. Then when I find them again at the local book sales I buy them again, and eventually hand them out to someone else who asks.

Keep up the great work, and I hope you are feeling well.
—P. L.

. . . . . .

Hello there,

I don't actually have a question. I just wanted to thank Mr. Diamond so very, very much. I am thirty-nine now, but was first introduced to *Fit For Life* almost twenty years ago. I just wanted to say thank you for giving me and so many others, FFL. It's not just some diet and exercise program. FFL gives anyone who is willing to accept it all of the tools they will ever need to love and nurture themselves. In times like these where families are often broken and support is often lacking, so many of us have not been taught how to cherish ourselves. FFL offers up to anyone willing to listen, the gift of self and that's huge. That's priceless.

Thank you, Mr. Diamond for your work, for the strength of your convictions, and for sharing all of that with all of us. You are saving so many lives, mine included, and I'm just so thankful.
—T. H.

. . . . . .

Hello,

I just finished my first Harvey Diamond book and my life will be forever changed. I plan to read all his books now and when my children are at this reading level, I will pass the books on to them to read. I am so grateful for Harvey Diamond and this book. I don't need a piece of paper to see that this book is brilliant!!! I know it is! I am recommending this to everyone I can think of and then some.

God bless Harvey Diamond and thank you from the very depths of my soul. Your book has changed my life and how I view my life, my body, and my health.

Kindest Regards,

—S. K.

* * * * *

Dear Harvey,

I am honored to share my success story: lost weight; menopause symptoms diminished; TMJ syndrome pain gone; more energy; and better sleep! I am fifty-one years old and I feel better than I have in years! I had great success in the late 80s with *Fit For Life*! Over the years, I moved away from the plan, tried the usual fad diets, ended up confused and actually gained weight. A few months ago, I came to my senses and went back to what made sense: fruits and vegetables, food combining, and *Fit For Life*! I have lost thirty pounds and feel great! Thank you,

—P. P.

* * * * *

Hi!

I am so thankful for coming across Harvey Diamond's *Fit For Life* book in 1986 when I was twenty-eight. At that time I was suffering with chronic constipation, heartburn every day and night since I was eight years old, no energy, and depression. My nervous system was out of whack. I knew this couldn't be right for a twenty-eight-year-old to be experiencing. The *Fit For Life* book was the only thing that made so much sense to me, so I decided to try it. Thank God I did because now twenty years later I feel better than I did when I was eighteen years old. Most of the people I know that are my age, forty-eight, are suffering with pain or some type of ailment. I was never overweight but my weight has stayed the same for twenty years, even after going

through menopause, and I look like I did twenty years ago. No one has ever been able to guess my age. Thank you, Harvey!
—J. S.

. . . . .

To Whom it May Concern,

My wife had stage 3 colon cancer and the doctors gave her a 20 to 30 percent chance to live five years. After reading Harvey's book *Fit For Life: A New Beginning,* she opted not to have chemotherapy. The doctors were upset after her decision, but after just six months no cancer traces were found!

Now after many CT scans and multiple blood works completed, she has no doubt that she made the right decision, and after just a few months she returned to work and feels great! (She was previously hospitalized for fifty-seven days and had an in-home nurse three to four days per week due to complications).

Today no one believes she has ever been sick. Also, my doctor has taken me off blood pressure meds after fourteen years!

Thank you, Harvey, from our whole heart and keep up the fight!
—M. B.

. . . . .

Dearest Mr. Diamond,

I just wasn't going to let another day go by without saying how much I appreciate your taking your time to call my son-in-law last evening. I cannot begin to express enough my deepest gratitude to you. Just for your caring enough to call, has given him the "boost" he so eminently needs at this "crossover" in his life. The ability to speak directly with you personally has brought so much encouragement and hope to him, as well as my daughter too. It is indescribable.

I truly believe with all my heart that your unselfish devotion to mankind is a blessing from God. Am I giving too much praise? I don't think so! You deserve so much more. You have said many times in your books that there comes a time when we must lean on our own understanding and "good common sense" against those that have indoctrinated us with the incorrect way to take care of our own health issues; but not so often are we strong enough to do so without the aid and encouragement that you've brought this humble little family of ours by your call and emails to us personally.

You cannot possibly know how much you're appreciated by us and you'll never know how much you have affected my family's lives as well as mine. Just believe me when I tell you, YOU HAVE! I only wish my mom was here to have enjoyed this special time of my life. She would be proud!

Thank you once again, Harvey Diamond, for you kindness. You are a wonderful human being. God bless you and long life to you.
—G. S.

Appendix

Dr. Steven Lamm
on The Role of
Enzymes in Weight Loss

Dr. Steven Lamm is a practicing internist and faculty member at New York University School of Medicine. Known to millions as the house doctor on ABC-TV's The View, *Dr. Lamm regularly offers his analyses and comments on a wide variety of health and medical-related topics on television and radio. He is the author or coauthor of several popular books including the best seller* Thinner at Last *and his latest book,* No Guts, No Glory! *A graduate of Columbia University and New York University School of Medicine, Dr. Lamm is the recipient of numerous honors and awards. He is active in clinical research and is a panel physician for the New York State Athletic Commission. Passionate about good digestion and enzyme therapy, Dr. Lamm combines his impressive education and experience with down-to-earth solutions for good digestive health.*

Dr. Lamm has most graciously agreed to provide some further information on enzymes in general and specifically the ingredients that make up the Slender GR™ *enzyme.*

When I was approached about contributing material for Harvey Diamond's new book, I must admit, I was honored to have the opportunity to contribute. I have seen firsthand how enzymes can change lives. This is not an exaggeration; they can change lives; enzymes are the energy of life. As already mentioned earlier by Harvey in this book, enzymes are responsible for all life on earth and without them all life would cease to exist. They play a critical role in digesting foods, delivering nutrients to the cells, and detoxification. Though each of these processes is essential for good health, one must also maintain his or her optimal weight in order to fully benefit from improving these efficiencies with enzyme supplements.

Harvey has asked me to discuss how the enzyme blend Glucoreductase™ works within the body to produce benefits in supporting weight loss and maintaining your ideal weight. It has been clear to me from my thirty years of practice that obesity is a complex biological condition that takes more than just will power to conquer. Glucoreductase™ can be a useful adjunct to a good nutritional program and exercise.

GLUCOREDUCTASE™

Glucoreductase™ offers a unique approach to weight loss that has a biologic basis for it. Glucoreductase™ is a combination of several enzymes. Two of the main ingredients in the blend are the enzymes lipase and transglucosidase. Lipase is the enzyme that breaks down fat. It stands to reason that if a person is able to fully digest the fat in their diet, they will store less of it.

Though lipase is a crucial part of this blend, transglucosidasen plays an equally important role. Transglucosidase is a plant-based enzyme with unusual characteristics. Research suggests that the enzyme transglucosidase changes starch (carbohydrate) to a form that is less likely to be absorbed and less likely to cause a rise in blood sugar and insulin following a meal. In addition, it happens to produce a substance called an oligosaccharide that is helpful to our important gut bacteria.

When Glucoreductase™ is in the presence of starchy carbohydrates it uses them to build non-soluble fiber. Digestive enzymes break down starchy carbohydrates into simple sugars, which are utilized for energy and are also stored as fat. Glucoreductase™ uses these simple sugars to build what is called oligosaccharides or fiber.

This fiber is not utilized as energy nor is it stored as fat, rather it travels through the intestinal tract and provides a food source to the beneficial bacteria that reside there.

I have been frustrated at the paucity of the pharmaceuticals that are available and welcome a nutraceutical that I can suggest to patients in their battle of the bulge. The only nutraceutical I am aware of that contains Glucoreductase™ is Slender GR™ by Enzymedica.

OBESITY AND BLOOD SUGAR

Starchy carbohydrates we chew and swallow are broken down by digestive enzymes into simple sugars; one of the sugars it produces is called glucose. Glucose is essential for energy; in fact it is one of our best sources of energy and is beneficial to the body. However, too much glucose in the blood is bad, it can literally kill us! To protect us from this, the pancreas produces a hormone called insulin. Insulin reduces glucose in the blood by causing glucose to be taken up by the muscle and fat tissue (adipose tissue). In other words, a high demand for insulin creates an environment perfect for storing large amounts of fat. This causes people to gain weight and it makes it increasingly difficult to lose weight. Glucoreductase™, by converting some simple sugars into fiber, succeeds in lowering demand and output of insulin. Incidentally, what I have just described is also the biggest contributor to type-2 diabetes and pre-diabetes.

PILOT STUDIES ON GLUCOREDUCTASE™

There are a couple of interesting studies funded by Enzymedica, which have been conducted that support the efficacy of Slender GR™.

In the first pilot, there were twenty-one participants. The length of the study was just thirty days and the individuals were instructed not to change anything in their diet or lifestyle. They consumed two capsules of Slender GR™ with each meal. The results were impressive. The participants reported:

❏ Increase in energy levels and improved digestion (40% described unanticipated benefits including improved digestion and energy levels)

❏ A decrease in weekly weight (50% lost an average of 4 pounds in 30 days)

❏ An improvement in how their clothes fit (40% felt that their clothes fit better)

With this information, Enzymedica made some additional improvements to the formula. With the same instructions, the second group of ten participants reported similar results as above with a couple of important differences:

❏ 70% lost an average of 8 pounds (30% lost 10 pounds or more)

• • •

What makes these results especially impressive is that all participants were told not to change the way they eat. Usually this type of research on a product is accompanied by a strict diet. Keep in mind that the only FDA approved over-the-counter "weight-loss" product is ALLI. The weight-loss results expected from taking ALLI is 3–5 pounds of additional weight-loss *PER YEAR* when combined with diet and exercise! Also of note is that Enzymedica funded a study prior to the weight-loss pilot studies to determine the effects a separate version of the product had on blood sugar. The participants experienced an average decrease of 30% in the rise of their blood sugar when challenged by a sugary sweet. The results were published in the *American Journal of Translational Research*.

As you can no doubt tell, I am very excited about the role enzymes play in maintaining a healthy weight. I am currently undergoing trials with this enzyme blend in helping patients control their weight and modify their blood sugar and insulin levels.

Once again, I wish to thank Harvey for the opportunity to provide this information.

INDEX

About the Author

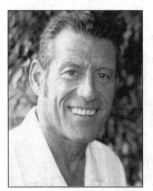 Harvey Diamond is one of the most celebrated and successful health authors in history, certainly one of today's truly great health thinkers.

He has been studying and teaching the principles of healthful living for more than 35 years and is recognized as one of the most effective and well-respected authors on the subject of health in the world. He is considered to be one of the original pioneers credited with helping shift people toward a healthier eating lifestyle.

Owing to his forward thinking, innovative approach to health and well-being his Fit For Life books have sold over 12 million copies in 33 languages and are read in over 80 countries. He has helped millions of people worldwide to not only dramatically improve their health, but also to overcome serious, catastrophic disease, including cancer.

The original Fit For Life book was only one of four books to sell 2 million hardcover copies in the entire decade of the 1980s and was fourth in total U.S. non-fiction sales in that decade. The book continued to break records in the 1990s, is still in high demand on Amazon and still sells 100,000 copies a year worldwide. It held the #1 position on the prestigious New York Times Bestseller list for an unprecedented 40 consecutive weeks, and held bestseller status in *USA Today, Time Magazine, the Los Angeles Times Book Review, Publishers Weekly* and the *San Francisco Chronicle Review,* to name only a few. In 1986 it achieved the coveted position on the *Publisher's Weekly* Top 25 Bestselling Books in Publishing History List, along with *Gone with the Wind* and the Bible.

During this time, Harvey made multiple appearances on *Oprah Winfrey, Larry King, Phil Donahue, Nightline, Geraldo Rivera, Merv Griffin, The Regis and Kathy Lee Show, Good Morning America, The Today Show, Sally Jesse Raphael, QVC, Pat Robertson's 700 Club,* and many others. Introducing his appearance on *ABC's Nightline with Ted Koppel,* it was stated that his book was the fastest selling book of its kind in history.

Fit For Life spawned juice and salad bars, and the juicing industry. It was a pivotal force in the advent of the natural food supermarket and the explosion of natural food consumption nationwide. The book was a trigger for Surgeon General Koop's New Dietary Guidelines for the American people and launched a nutritional awakening in the United States and other Western countries.

Harvey triumphed over a devastating condition called Peripheral Neuropathy, brought on by Agent Orange poisoning while serving his country in Vietnam. Although he has significant lingering damage to his musculature, thanks to his considerable understanding of the human body and its proper care, he is one of the longest-known survivors of this devastating condition to still be walking around on his own without assistance. Despite his physical challenges, Harvey is as positive, upbeat, and good-natured a person as you will ever meet. He is an inspiration to all who meet him.

A primary reason for Harvey Diamond's phenomenal success lies not only in his ability to simplify seemingly complicated subjects with commonsense information that helps people, but it is also his engaging writing style. His style is conversational and totally non-technical. In his words, "I don't write for doctors and scientists. I write for folks. You won't need a dictionary by your side in order to understand what you read."

His words seem to come alive and jump right off the page at you. His reader-friendly, light-hearted, frequently humorous approach to writing make many a reader comment that, "It's almost as though he's sitting in your living room having a conversation with you. It reads more like a novel than a health book."

Contact Information

To stay in touch with Harvey Diamond and obtain more information about the *Weight Loss Enzyme* Slender GR™, *Digestive Enzymes*, services, newsletter, or Social Network Sites, the official contact points are as follows:

Website
www.harveydiamond.com
www.vpnutrition.com
www.fitforlifetime.com

Email
info@harveydiamond.com
info@vpnutrition.com

Facebook
www.facebook.com/harveydiamond

Twitter
www.twitter.com/harveydiamond

Follow Harvey on his Blog
www.harveydiamond.info

Telephone
877-335-1509 / 941-966-9727

Postal Address
Harvey Diamond
P.O. Box 811, Osprey, Florida 34229

Phillip C. DeMio, M.D.
Executive Director, American Medical Autism Board
320 Orchardview Avenue, Suite #2
Seven Hills, Ohio 44131
Website: www.drdemio.com
Ph. 216-901-0441
Fax-216-901-0485

Steven Lamm, M.D.
12 East 86th Street
New York, N.Y. 10028

Dr. M. Mamadou
Phytomedic Labs, LLC
Ph. 800-246-1827

Natalia KW Recipes
Website: www.NataliaKW.com
E-mail: lifestyle@nataliakw.com
Facebook: http://www.facebook.com/PureNataliaKW

Toby Coriell
Autism Hope Alliance Enzyme Science /
Medical Professional Use Enzymes
Ph. 941-966-9727 / 877-335-1509
Website: www.vpnutrition.com
E-mail: info@vpnutrition.com